HEMOLYTIC UREMIC SYNDROME

SYMPTOMS, TREATMENT OPTIONS AND PROGNOSIS

RENAL AND UROLOGIC DISORDERS

Additional books in this series can be found on Nova's website under the Series tab.

Additional e-books in this series can be found on Nova's website under the e-book tab.

HEMOLYTIC UREMIC SYNDROME

SYMPTOMS, TREATMENT OPTIONS AND PROGNOSIS

GLENNA CLAYTON
EDITOR

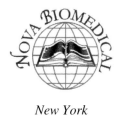

New York

Library of Congress Cataloging-in-Publication Data

ISBN: 978-1-63463-227-0

Library of Congress Control Number: 2014952255

Published by Nova Science Publishers, Inc. † New York

Contents

Preface

Hemolytic uremic syndrome (HUS) is characterized by the triad non-immune micro-angiopathic hemolytic anemia, thrombocytopenia and acute renal failure. The disease mainly affects children one to ten years of age. It begins after an incubation period of 4 to 7 days with abrupt onset of bloody diarrhea and abdominal pain. Two to ten days later, microangiopathy, haemolytic anaemia, thrombocytopenia, and acute renal failure develop. HUS microangiopathy can involve almost any organ, but damage to kidneys and central nervous system cause the most severe clinical problems. This book discusses the symptoms, the treatment options and prognosis of HUS.

Chapter I – The interplay between inflammation and thrombosis in the pathophysiology and treatment of hemolytic uremic syndrome (HUS) is an emerging paradigm. Several lines of clinical and laboratory evidence implicate thrombin activation in multiple, if not all, forms of thrombotic microangiopathies (TMAs). Accumulating evidence indicates that thrombin mediates both inflammatory and prothrombotic effects in TMAs. The endothelium is a key factor in inflammation and thrombosis. Endothelial cells (ECs) are well-established regulators of hemostasis. EC hemostatic regulatory mechanisms include the coagulation cascade initiated by tissue factor binding factor VII, regulation of fibrinolysis by endothelial expression of tissue plasminogen activator (tPA) and plasminogen activator inhibitor type 1 (PAI-1), and anticoagulant functions of the thrombomodulin-protein C pathway. Newer evidence establishing endothelium as a regulator of inflammation includes the function of thrombomodulin in regulating complement activation and anaphylatoxin degradation. Endothelial exposure to Shiga toxin results in the hallmark feature of microvascular thrombosis. Whether thrombosis results from endothelial perturbation and procoagulant changes or cell death and subsequent thrombosis remains unclear. In either case, thrombin activation may be a central factor. When considering therapeutic strategies for TMAs, a fundamental distinction should be made between endothelial cell perturbation and cell death. EC perturbation suggests the possibility of therapeutic interventions aimed at restoring normal physiology, whereas different strategies may be required to manage the thrombotic consequences of EC death. The modulation of thrombin activity may offer new effective strategies in the treatment of TMAs.

Chapter II – Since the mid 1970s, membrane modules became available, plasma separation techniques have gained in importance in the past few years. The advantages of this method are a complete separation of the corpuscular components from the plasma and due to increased blood flow rate higher efficacy. Furthermore, cell damage – especially to thrombocytes – occurs less using membranes than centrifuges for cell separation. In this time the demand for treatments of children and adolescents was increasing more and more. The problem was to win the industry to minmize the hollow fibers, the tubes, the extracorporeal blood volume and at last the machine. The use of therapeutic apheresis (TA) in pediatric patients has always been restricted by technical difficulties and the low incidence of diseases requiring this kind of treatment. The development of new, more sophisticated membranes has allowed to new techniques. The adsorption technologies allow the most selective separation of plasma components without the use of substitution solutions. Based on many years of experience with extracorporeal circulation in end-stage renal disease, the authors try to give an overview of TA in renal diseases. TA has been successfully introduced in a variety of autoantibody-mediated diseases. The updated information on immunology and molecular biology of different renal diseases are discussed in relation to the rationale for apheresis therapy and its place in combination with other modern treatments. The different renal diseases can be treated by various apheresis methods such as therapeutic plasma exchange (TPE) with substitution solution, or with online plasma or blood purification using adsorption columns which contain biological or non biological agents. The following diseases are discussed: hemolytic uremic syndrome (HUS), rapidly progressive glomerulonephritis (RPGN), including anti-glomerular basement membrane antibody glomerulonephritis (anti-GBM RPGN), RPGN with or without glomerular deposition, pauci-immune PPGN, immune complex nephritis (ICN), and various glomerulonephritis with nephrotic syndrome (NS), myoglobulinemic renal failure, acute kidney injury (AKI), and kidney transplant rejection. Pathogenetical aspects are demonstrated in these diseases, in which they are clarified. TA has been shown to effectively remove the auto-antibodies from blood and lead to rapid clinical improvement. For the renal diseases which can be treated with TA the guidelines of the Apheresis Applications Committee (AAC) of the American Society for Apheresis (ASFA) are cited. The aim of the present review is to describe the solutions adopted to solve technical difficulties related to priming, vascular access and monitoring and then to evaluate clinical results.

Chapter III – Atypical HUS (aHUS) is a sub-type of Hemolytic Uremic Syndrome in which the origin of the thrombotic micro-angiopathy (TMA) is the result of a decreased regulation of the alternative complement pathway on cell surfaces due to a genetic cause. aHUS is a rare disease that, despite the standard treatment with plasmapheresis, often progresses to terminal renal failure with associated co-morbidity, such as long term renal replacement therapy (RRT). As such, aHUS has a poor prognosis and is associated with high morbidity and mortality. The complement system plays a key role in the induction of endothelial damage in patients with aHUS. Recent advances in genetic research demonstrate that mutations in the genes that code for complement factors provoke the induction of endothelial damage. The observation that excessive activation of the alternative pathway of complement underlies the pathogenesis of aHUS seems to make clear that the complement inhibition is the crux of the treatment. Eculizumab (Soliris®) is a monoclonal antibody (anti-C5) that inhibits the terminal fraction of the complement system, by blocking the formation of a cell membrane attack complex and C5a. It is well known that eculizumab involves an interruption of the TMA process. Eculizumab was first introduced as treatment of paroxysmal nocturnal hemoglobinuria and seemed also effective in the treatment of plasmapheresis resistant aHUS. Therefore, in 2011 both the US Food and Drug Administration (FDA) and the European Medicines Agency (EMA) approved the use of eculizumab to treat aHUS. Eculizumab improves renal function not only in early treated patients without need of RRT, but also in patients with RRT, which implies an improvement of health related quality of life. In other words, eculizumab should be initiated as early as feasible in order to optimize the recovery of renal function, and should also be used in patients after renal transplantation when it seems certain that an underlying aHUS could relapse. In contrast, Soliris® should be permanently recommended to patients, unless discontinuation of Soliris® is clinically indicated. However, therapy with Soliris® is expensive and the administration is subject to several conditions. Eculizumab is not without risks, being associated with the development of meningococcal disease. That means all patients should be vaccinated before the onset of treatment and should in addition receive prophylactic antibiotics. Furthermore, a lifetime intake of immunosuppressive therapy has a

considerable impact on a patient's quality of life. To conclude, the
administration of eculizumab has serious advantages for a patient's personal
life and social interest in general.

Chapter IV – HUS is defined by the triad of haemolytic anaemia, acute
renal failure, and thrombocytopenia. It became a public health problem
following the European outbreak of E. coli (O104:H4) gastroenteritis in 2011.
The disease mainly affects children one to 10 years of age. It begins after an
incubation period of 4 to 7 days with abrupt onset of bloody diarrhea and
abdominal pain. Two to ten days later, microangiopathy, haemolytic anaemia,
thrombocytopenia, and acute renal failure develop. HUS microangiopathy can
involve almost any organ, but damage to kidneys and central nervous system
cause the most severe clinical problems. HUS is classified into three primary
types: (1) HUS due to infections, often associated with diarrhea (D+HUS),
with the rare exception of HUS due to a severe disseminated infection caused
by Streptococcus; (2) HUS related to complement abnormalities, such HUS is
also known as "atypical HUS" and is not diarrhea associated (D-HUS); and (3)
HUS of unknown etiology that usually occurs in the course of systemic
diseases or physiopathologic conditions such as pregnancy.

In: Hemolytic Uremic Syndrome
Editors: Glenna Clayton

ISBN: 978-1-63463-227-0
© 2015 Nova Science Publishers, Inc.

Chapter I

The Role of Thrombin in Hemolytic Uremic Syndrome and Other Thrombotic Microangiopathies

William Nicholas Rose[1], Kenneth D. Friedman[2]
and Thomas J. Raife[1]
[1]Department of Pathology and Laboratory Medicine,
University of Wisconsin School of Medicine and Public Health,
Madison, Wisconsin, US
[2]Blood Research Institute, Blood Center of Wisconsin,
Milwaukee, Wisconsin, US

Abstract

The interplay between inflammation and thrombosis in the pathophysiology and treatment of hemolytic uremic syndrome (HUS) is an emerging paradigm. Several lines of clinical and laboratory evidence implicate thrombin activation in multiple, if not all, forms of thrombotic microangiopathies (TMAs). Accumulating evidence indicates that thrombin mediates both inflammatory and prothrombotic effects in TMAs.

The endothelium is a key factor in inflammation and thrombosis. Endothelial cells (ECs) are well-established regulators of hemostasis. EC hemostatic regulatory mechanisms include the coagulation cascade initiated by tissue factor binding factor VII, regulation of fibrinolysis by endothelial expression of tissue plasminogen activator (tPA) and plasminogen activator inhibitor type 1 (PAI-1), and anticoagulant functions of the thrombomodulin-protein C pathway. Newer evidence establishing endothelium as a regulator of inflammation includes the function of thrombomodulin in regulating complement activation and anaphylatoxin degradation. Endothelial exposure to Shiga toxin results in the hallmark feature of microvascular thrombosis. Whether thrombosis results from endothelial perturbation and procoagulant changes or cell death and subsequent thrombosis remains unclear. In either case, thrombin activation may be a central factor.

When considering therapeutic strategies for TMAs, a fundamental distinction should be made between endothelial cell perturbation and cell death. EC perturbation suggests the possibility of therapeutic interventions aimed at restoring normal physiology, whereas different strategies may be required to manage the thrombotic consequences of EC death. The modulation of thrombin activity may offer new effective strategies in the treatment of TMAs.

Introduction

This chapter addresses the role of thrombin regulation in the pathophysiology of HUS and other TMAs, such as thrombotic thrombocytopenic purpura (TTP) and atypical hemolytic syndrome (aHUS). Highlighted topics include: the role of thrombin in normal EC physiology; thrombin modulation in disease states; the effects of Shiga toxin on thrombin generation; the interaction between thrombin and ECs; therapeutic strategies that target thrombin and thrombin regulation; and the intersection of inflammation and thrombosis in TMA.

1. Thrombin Activation in Endothelial Cell Physiology

TMA is a final common pathway of many disease states. TMAs are most consistently manifested by platelet and fibrin microthrombi resulting from a wide variety of etiologies. Etiologies can be as disparate as Shiga toxin which preferentially targets renal endothelium in HUS, autoantibodies against the hemostatic regulatory enzyme ADAMTS13 in TTP, and congenital defects of complement regulatory factors in aHUS. Microvascular thrombosis typically leads to thrombocytopenia and mechanical hemolysis as well as other signs and symptoms that vary depending on the etiology. [1] In clinical medicine, an appreciation of the underlying etiology of TMA is vital for the selection of rational therapies that are tailored to the specific defects. [2-4]

Many lines of evidence have shown that TMAs are characterized by significant changes in ECs. [5] ECs perform critical roles in hemostasis, inflammation, and wound healing. [6] Thrombin generation and regulation are two of many functions influenced by ECs. [7] Additional functions include the regulation of vascular tone, selective infiltration and adhesion of leukocytes, promotion of clotting, and prevention of spontaneous clot formation. The key mechanisms by which ECs regulate hemostasis are briefly reviewed below. Recent comprehensive reviews have been published. [8]

Procoagulant Mediators

ECs regulate hemostasis by providing access to context-specific mediators. [9] Two key procoagulants are von Willebrand factor (vWF) and tissue factor (TF), which are utilized for physiologic clot formation when damage to ECs results in exposure of blood to subendothelial tissues. [10] Platelet adhesion mediated by vWF is typically the first step of clot formation. Circulating and EC-secreted vWF binds to exposed collagen and tethers circulating platelets. Further platelet accumulation occurs via the mechanisms underlying platelet aggregation as the coagulation cascade is activated, and fibrin is formed on or about the surfaces of platelets. [11]

The coagulation cascade is initiated by TF. [12] While ECs do not express prothrombotic amounts of transmembrane TF on their surfaces under resting conditions, subendothelial cells express TF on their surfaces in large quantities. [13] When TF binds to circulating factor VII on a phospholipid surface in the presence of calcium ions, the coagulation cascade is activated, which leads to the conversion of prothrombin to thrombin and, consequently, fibrinogen to fibrin. [14] Normal ECs serve as a barrier to prevent the binding of vWF to collagen and the binding of factor VII to subendothelial TF. When activated, ECs release vWF and express TF on their surfaces.

Anticoagulant Mediators

The primary function of anticoagulants expressed by normal ECs under physiologic conditions is to prevent unnecessary clot formation. Three important EC anticoagulants are tissue factor pathway inhibitor (TFPI), heparan sulfate, and thrombomodulin. TFPI is produced primarily by ECs and inhibits the TF-factor VIIa complex. [15] Heparan sulfate is expressed on the surface of ECs and is a cofactor for the protease inhibitor antithrombin, a potent inactivator of thrombin. [16, 17] Thrombomodulin is largely produced by ECs and indirectly promotes the inactivation of factors Va and VIIIa. [18] The inactivation of factors Va and VIIIa occurs in a multistep process: Endothelial protein C receptor (EPCR) secures circulating anticoagulant protein C to the EC surface. Thrombomodulin expressed on EC surfaces binds thrombin to form a complex that catalyzes the activation of protein C to form activated protein C (aPC). aPC and its cofactor protein S cleave factors Va and VIIIa into inactive forms. [19] The disruption of the clotting cascade by inactivation of factors Va and VIIIa downregulates thrombin production.

Profibrinolytic and Antifibrinolytic Mediators

While not strictly part of either clot formation or anticoagulation, fibrinolysis is a vital component of hemostasis as it helps ensure appropriate clot size, strength, and eventual dissolution. [20] Plasmin, derived from its circulating inactive form, plasminogen, is the primary enzyme that breaks down polymers of both fibrin and fibrinogen in the process of fibrinolysis. [21] D-dimer is one degradation product of fibrinolysis. Mediators involved in the fibrinolytic system include the profibrinolytic enzymes urokinase-type plasminogen activators (uPAs) and tissue plasminogen activator (tPA), and the antifibrinolytic factors PAI-1 and α_2-plasmin inhibitor (α_2-PI).

Plasmin that is generated from plasminogen on the cell surface is largely sheltered from inhibitors. Plasminogen receptors are expressed on platelets and all nucleated cells, particularly ECs. uPAs and tPA are released by stimulated ECs, as well as by granulocytes and monocytes as acute phase reactants. These uPAs and tPA enhance the conversion of cell-surface plasminogen to plasmin.

Circulating PAI-1 binds to uPAs and tPA and inhibits the activation of plasminogen to plasmin. [22] Circulating α_2-PI directly inhibits circulating plasmin and also impairs the binding of plasmin and plasminogen to fibrin clots. [23] In addition, α_2-PI secreted by platelets prevents excessive fibrinolysis.

In addition to its critical role in hemostasis, plasmin is a potent inhibitor the complement cascade at the level of C3 and C5. [24] Conversely, plasmin has been shown to stimulate proinflammatory cytokines and cell signaling pathways. It has been postulated that chronic inflammatory and immune diseases may be explained in part by increased plasmin activity. [25]

In summary, ECs are intimately involved in the regulation of hemostasis and thrombosis through many pathways. The following section will emphasize how disease states lead to changes in EC thrombin regulation.

2. Modulation of Thrombin in TMAs

The equilibrium maintained by normally functioning ECs may be disrupted by disease. A recently appreciated central concept in the field of endothelial cell biology is that ECs are heterogeneous and dynamic rather than homogeneous and inert. [26-29] Under normal conditions, ECs strike a balance between procoagulant and anticoagulant influences in an uneven and localized manner, depending on the location in the body. When ECs are stimulated, the balance is usually tipped toward a more procoagulant function, presumably to prevent hemorrhage.

Inflammatory cytokines such as tumor necrosis factor-alpha (TNF-α) and interleukin-1 (IL-1) are among the most common factors that stimulate ECs to express a more prothrombotic phenotype. While this procoagulant EC response may be an appropriate response to an insult, it can also result in life-threatening or limb-threatening thrombosis.

A number of lines of evidence implicate a role of EC injury and thrombin production in disease states. In vitro studies have shown that IL-1 is a potent inducer of a TF-like substance in ECs. [30] In addition, ECs exposed to IL-1 exhibit decreased tPA activity and increased PAI-1 activity. [31, 32] These in vitro observations suggest that an inflammatory stimulus can induce a procoagulant, antifibrinolytic state in the vasculature.

The relevance of this model of EC perturbation in TMA is supported by historical studies of TTP showing increased thrombin production and activity as well as impaired fibrinolysis. [33, 34] Plasminogen activator was observed to be absent in TTP microthrombi compared to uninvolved vessels, [35] and inhibition of tPA and decreased tPA function were demonstrated. [36] The specificity of this hypofibrinolytic condition in TMA syndromes was further supported by observations of elevated PAI-1 in the acute stage of TTP, which occurred at levels well beyond those seen in patients with disseminated intravascular coagulation. [37]

Many studies have demonstrated downregulation of the thrombomodulin-protein C pathway in a variety of inflammatory and thrombotic conditions. [38-46] The likely involvement of this EC pathway in HUS and TMAs will be discussed at greater length below.

In summary, many inflammatory conditions and factors have been shown to alter EC regulation of hemostatic pathways to produce a prothrombotic, hypofibrinolytic state. From this framework, the pathological role of Shiga toxin in HUS will be discussed.

3. Effects of Shiga Toxin on Endothelial Cells and Thrombin Production

Having established that normal EC regulation of hemostatic pathways can be modulated in disease states, the following section addresses the roles of EC injury and thrombin production in HUS and other TMAs.

Endothelial Cell States

Endothelial cell states can be placed on a conceptual spectrum from least to most perturbed: resting, activated, chronically activated, damaged/injured, and dead. [47] Intermediate distinctions may overlap, and each broad category has many subtypes (reversible vs. irreversible activation, and death by apoptosis vs. necrosis). [48] Most of the EC changes that were previously discussed stop short of cell death. Thus, a relatively broad yet clear distinction can be made between sub-lethal EC perturbations and insults that lead to EC death. In HUS, many studies have established that EC activation, injury, and death, and the resulting microvascular thrombosis, are consequences of the damage done by Shiga toxin. The remainder of this section will address studies that emphasize the specific roles of thrombin and ECs in HUS. The mechanisms of EC injury and thrombosis resulting from Shiga toxin may also apply generally to the complement-mediated injury of aHUS.

Thrombin Generation in HUS

The renal lesion characteristic of HUS includes intracapillary glomerular fibrin deposition. [49] This fibrin deposition can be divided into two phases: the formation of circulating fibrin complexes and its deposition in the glomerular capillaries. The first phase has been successfully inhibited in animal models and in vitro with anticoagulants, while the second stage has not. [50]

Since thrombin activation and fibrin clot production are principal components of Shiga toxin EC injury, a rational treatment strategy might be the administration of anticoagulants. However, most clinical studies have shown little efficacy of anticoagulation treatments in HUS. The lack of efficacy of anticoagulation treatment may be because the thrombi have already formed and the damage has been done by the time the syndrome becomes manifest. Despite the lack of success so far, future treatment strategies will have to address this pathogenic process.

Effects of Shiga Toxin on ECs and Thrombin Activation

Shiga toxin binding and induction of renal EC injury is the primary inciting pathogenic event in HUS. [51] The EC injury leads to platelet adhesion and aggregation together with fibrin thrombus formation. Shiga toxin has been shown to stimulate thrombin activation by ECs via four often overlapping pathways: cellular activation, apoptosis, necrosis, and complement activation. When injury is severe, subendothelial collagen is exposed, platelets adhere and aggregate, and ECs lose their antithrombotic properties.

In addition to direct EC damage, Shiga toxin can cause ECs to lose their normal thromboresistant phenotype. [52] Prothrombotic EC abnormalities precede clinical evidence of renal damage. [53] EC procoagulant changes are mediated by inflammatory pathways. Shiga toxin can cause EC activation and cytokine release as well as cell death. [54] The sub-lethal injury process in ECs involves a ribotoxic stress response, upregulation of adhesion molecules for leukocytes, and promotion of a prothrombotic state. [55] The inflammatory response, mainly in the form of cytokine release, leads to further prothrombotic changes. Shiga toxin works in concert with TNF-α or IL-1β to induce a cytotoxic effect on ECs, [54] and induced cytokines stimulate expression of TF on activated ECs. In addition to a shift toward a procoagulant phenotype, ECs have been shown to secrete large amounts of prothrombotic ultralarge vWF multimers after exposure to Shiga toxin. [56]

Inflammatory cytokines released from Shiga toxin-injured ECs inhibit the function of major anticoagulant pathways (antithrombin, protein C, and tissue factor pathway inhibitor). [57, 58] The prothrombotic state is compounded further by the inhibition of fibrinolysis resulting from cytokine-stimulated PAI-1 release in excess of tPA and uPAs. [59, 60] Finally, in addition to EC activation and injury, EC apoptotic cell death creates a prothrombotic stimulus by direct exposure of subendothelial TF and collagen.

In summary, Shiga toxin induces EC activation and injury leading to an inflammatory milieu and a prothrombotic phenotype. [61] The Shiga toxin model of TMA serves to illustrate the interplay between thrombosis and inflammation in TMA, and exemplifies the need to address these interrelated pathogenic processes in future treatment strategies. [55]

Effects of Thrombin on Endothelial Cells

Thrombin itself has cell stimulating properties. Thrombin signaling in ECs is mediated by protease-activated receptors (PARs). PAR-1 is the main thrombin receptor in ECs. [62, 63] Thrombin cleaves an external domain of PAR-1 leaving the remaining portion as a so-called tethered ligand that binds and activates the receptor. Once activated, PAR-1 interacts with a family of heterotrimeric G proteins and several subsequent signal intermediates. [64] These intermediates bind to an extensive variety of ligands that vary locally with the protein expression of the specific cell type. Thrombin signaling increases expression of many target genes that mediate cell proliferation, inflammation, leukocyte adhesion, vasomotor tone, and hemostasis. [64] Although the role of thrombin-mediated cell signaling in TMA is not well understood, it is likely that it contributes to EC injury.

4. Animal Models

Direct evaluation of histopathology in TMA patients is often limited by the risk of biopsy-associated bleeding complications. [65] Therefore, animal models have been exploited to gain insight into histopathological changes in TMAs, and to provide a model for experimentation. Although caution must be exercised in extrapolating findings to human medicine, animal models have provided critical observations about the TMA pathogenesis.

One important animal model of TTP pathophysiology is a genetically engineered ADAMTS13-deficient mouse. ADAMTS13 deficient mice develop and survive normally, overall. However, when these mice were challenged with Shiga toxin to induce endothelial cell injury, it caused systemic microvascular thrombosis resembling TTP. [66] The effect of Shiga toxin evoking a TMA syndrome in these otherwise healthy mice lacking ADAMTS13 suggested that endothelial cell injury is an essential component of TMA pathogenesis.

A similar experiment using mice that were deficient in both vWF and ADAMTS13 showed that the absence of vWF completely protects against Shiga toxin-induced thrombocytopenia. [67] These results demonstrated that vWF is required for the Shiga toxin-induced microvascular thrombosis, and the absence of TMA in this experiment suggests that the Shiga toxin caused EC stimulation rather than EC death. In other experiments using bacterial lipopolysaccharide, (LPS) rather than Shiga toxin, thrombocytopenia in mice was not altered by the absence of either vWF or ADAMTS13. These findings are more consistent with a severe EC injury from LPS resulting in coagulation-mediated thrombus formation. The authors posited that the LPS-induced thrombocytopenia may occur due to inflammatory processes rather than solely via an activation of coagulation.

An animal model that recapitulates the major aspects of human HUS was discovered in greyhound dogs. A naturally occurring disease known as idiopathic cutaneous and renal glomerular vasculopathy of greyhounds (CRVG) can develop after ingestion of enteropathic E. coli contaminated meat. The syndrome involves Shiga toxin-induced bloody diarrhea, ulcerating skin lesions, and acute renal failure. [68] The recognition of CRVG in greyhound kennels led to the development of an animal model in which administration of subcutaneous or intravenous of Shiga toxin results in rapid evolution of the CRVG syndrome.

The greyhound CRVG model was used to explore the role of thrombin in this HUS-like syndrome. In one study, dogs were anticoagulated with the direct thrombin inhibitor lepirudin *prior* to Shiga toxin challenge. [69] Of three dogs administered lepirudin prior to Shiga toxin, one developed CRVG while two were protected from developing the full syndrome. These two animals only showed hypersalivation and restlessness that quickly resolved. Moreover, hematological and biochemical parameters in the two surviving dogs were normal within 3 days. This study suggested that thrombin activity is a critical factor in the pathogenesis of HUS, and that early systemic thrombin inhibition might reduce or prevent its occurrence.

Since anticoagulation treatment after the onset of HUS has not been generally effective, it is unlikely that thrombin inhibition would be an effective treatment for established symptomatic HUS. However, an effective *preventive* strategy in patients at risk for developing HUS may warrant exploration. Much more extensive experimental work in animal models would be needed to refine such a strategy for human use.

Many in vitro and animal model studies implicate EC injury and thrombin generation as central factors in the development of HUS and other TMAs. While treatment strategies targeting thrombin activity face the obstacles of timing and bleeding risks, it is possible that future advances may yield more practical and effective approaches.

5. Treatments Targeting Thrombin in HUS and TMAs

The traditional view of inhibiting thrombin as a treatment for HUS is two-fold: 1) anticoagulation therapy is typically applied too late in the disease process, because much if not all of the damage has been done, and 2) empirical data show an overall increased risk of bleeding that is not offset by other clinical improvements. Several clinical investigations explored anticoagulation therapy for patients with HUS with unimpressive results. [70] While these clinical investigations should discourage further similar approaches to HUS treatment, promising options should remain under consideration.

Modulation of the Thrombomodulin-Protein C Pathway in Clinical Thrombosis

The discovery of thrombomodulin as a cofactor in the activation of protein C was a major advance in the understanding of thrombin regulation. Thrombomodulin expressed on EC surfaces binds thrombin and alters its substrate specificity, reducing its ability to cleave fibrinogen and increasing its ability to activate the anticoagulant protein C. [71, 72] The importance of thrombomodulin is evidenced by the procoagulant phenotype of transgenic mice that express thrombomodulin with reduced activity, and more dramatically by the embryonic lethality of deletion of the thrombomodulin gene in mice. [73-75]

In addition to its anticoagulant function, the thrombomodulin-protein C pathway has important anti-inflammatory functions. [76] Activated protein C binds to the endothelial protein C receptor (EPCR). This complex then activates PAR-1 on EC and other cells. PAR-1 signaling in ECs results in a cytoprotective effect. Activated protein C also downregulates apoptosis pathways in EC and neutralizes the cytotoxic effects of extracellular histones release from damaged cells. Administration of protein C in patients with severe protein C deficiency resolves both thrombotic and inflammatory lesions. [76]

Many lines of evidence have established that decreased expression or function of thrombomodulin plays a role in human thrombotic disorders. In vitro, EC thrombomodulin expression is downregulated by inflammatory factors that are relevant in thrombosis, such as endotoxin, homocysteine, and TNF-α. [39, 41, 44, 77] Inflammatory factors can also cleave thrombomodulin from EC surfaces and downregulate its function. [43, 78-80] In clinical studies, decreased EC expression or function of thrombomodulin has been associated with thrombotic conditions such as cardiovascular disease, stroke, and venous thromboembolism. [40, 81-83]

Clinical Observations: Activated Protein C

Therapeutic interventions have been explored involving augmentation of the thrombomodulin-protein C pathway to treat thrombotic disorders. Recent clinical studies have shown that infusion of recombinant soluble thrombomodulin has antithrombotic and possibly anti-inflammatory effects in the disseminated intravascular coagulation associated with acute promyelocytic leukemia (APL). [84-87] aPC has also been explored for its antithrombotic and anti-inflammatory effects. A pharmaceutical form of aPC was explored in clinical trials and marketed for the treatment of sepsis. Although initial clinical trials were promising, later analyses revealed increased bleeding risks and failed to show efficacy in reducing mortality. [88] The drug was withdrawn from the market, but the anticoagulant function of pharmaceutical aPC was demonstrated.

The possibility that decreased thrombomodulin expression contributes to microvascular thrombosis in HUS is indirectly supported by studies showing that the factor V Leiden mutation, which confers resistance to the anticoagulant effects of protein C, is overrepresented in a subset of TMA patients. [89, 90] More direct evidence of a possible role of thrombomodulin dysfunction in HUS is that stimulation of glomerular ECs with TNF-α and Shiga toxin 2 results in decreased thrombomodulin expression. [91] Moreover, elevated plasma thrombomodulin levels, indicative of cleavage from the EC surface, have been observed in both idiopathic and transplant-associated HUS. [92]

Clinical Observations: All-Trans Retinoic Acid

In the early 1990s, all-trans retinoic acid (ATRA) was introduced for the treatment of acute promyelocytic leukemia (APL). [93] The main therapeutic effect of ATRA is to stimulate the differentiation of APL cells into more mature myeloid forms. However, a striking adjunctive effect is the rapid resolution of the severe coagulopathy characteristic of APL. This resolution often occurs in advance of demonstrable APL cell differentiation. [94, 95] These observations led to the discovery that ATRA directly affects expression of thrombomodulin and TF by APL cells. ATRA downregulates TF expression and upregulates thrombomodulin expression independently of its effect on APL cell differentiation. [94, 96]

The anticoagulant-promoting properties of ATRA have been observed in ECs and other tissues that express thrombomodulin. [97] In ECs, ATRA upregulates expression of thrombomodulin and counteracts both the upregulation of TF and the downregulation of thrombomodulin that result from inflammatory cytokine stimulation. ATRA also promotes EC expression of tPA. [98-101] ATRA therefore counteracts prothrombotic inflammatory signals and stimulates expression of anticoagulant and profibrinolytic factors in ECs.

Retinoic Acid in TMA

Because of its marked antithrombotic effect in APL and in cell culture models, an oral form of retinoic acid has been used experimentally to treat TMA. In one case, a nine year-old African/Native American male presented with a history of headaches, nausea, vomiting and migratory joint pains. [102] His platelet count was 15,000/μL, and he had microangiopathic hemolytic anemia. He was treated with intravenous immunoglobulin and plasma infusion without resolution of his hematological abnormalities. Four weeks later his platelet count decreased to 4,000/µL, and he developed confusion and disorientation. He had proteinuria as well as elevated serum bilirubin and lactate dehydrogenase levels. He was diagnosed with TTP, received another dose of intravenous immunoglobulin, and was started on plasma exchange. He received 18 days of plasma exchange treatment after which heparin was added. His neurological symptoms resolved, but his hematological abnormalities remained. His neurological symptoms then reoccurred, and during the next 30 days he was treated with 18 staphylococcal protein A adsorption column procedures, two doses of vincristine, and splenectomy. His fever and hematological abnormalities persisted. His neurological abnormalities resolved and then recurred. He was then started on methylprednisone, and three days later, twice daily 13-*cis* retinoic acid. Within five days of starting oral retinoic acid treatment, his platelet count began to rise, and within 16 days, was within the normal range for the first time in over 60 days. The patient was discharged on twice-daily retinoic acid for six months and remained in remission throughout a two-year follow-up period.

In a second case, a 25-year-old female developed severe thrombocytopenia and microangiopathic hemolytic anemia following a respiratory illness. [103] Serum bilirubin levels and lactate dehydrogenase were elevated. Coagulation studies and ADAMTS13 levels were normal. The patient was diagnosed with "idiopathic TTP" and plasma exchange and corticosteroids were initiated. Despite these treatments, she developed hemiparesis and coma and her hemolysis and thrombocytopenia worsened. She was treated with vincristine and the platelet count began to rise. Soon thereafter, the platelet count dropped to severely low levels and hemolysis increased. Another dosage of vincristine was administered, and on day 22 of her hospital course she began a course of twice-daily 13-*cis* retinoic acid. Within three days of initiating retinoic acid treatment, her platelet count normalized and her hemoglobin began to increase. She was discharged eleven days later and remained on retinoic acid treatment for six months without relapse.

These two cases involving 13-*cis* retinoic acid as well as the impressive clinical efficacy of ATRA and soluble thrombomodulin in the treatment of the coagulopathy of APL provide rationale for therapeutic approaches aimed at augmenting thrombomodulin function in the treatment of HUS and other TMAs.

6. Inflammation and Thrombosis: Connections and Convergence

The emerging understanding of the intimate relationship between coagulation and inflammation is illustrated by a number of conditions. [104] Sepsis-associated and APL-associated disseminated intravascular coagulation (DIC) are two well-known examples. With regard to TMAs, the coincidence of pregnancy and obesity with episodes of TTP has been recognized for decades. [105, 106] The recognition that both pregnancy and obesity represent a spectrum of inflammatory conditions strongly suggests an inflammatory component in the pathogenesis of TMAs. [107] In addition, many studies demonstrate the ability of acute phase reactants to cause EC perturbation and TF upregulation. [47, 108-111] In TMA, the acute phase reactants procalcitonin and C-reactive protein (CRP) were dramatically elevated in a subset of patients with a TTP-like illness. [112] In ADAMTS13-deficient patients, elevated levels of CRP correlated directly with refractory disease as measured by longer treatment response times. [113] Thus, both inflammatory and hemostatic factors appear to be important in the pathogenesis and potentially the targeted treatment of TMAs.

The emerging discovery of the association between congenital defects in complement regulatory factors and atypical HUS (aHUS) underscores the interplay between thrombosis and inflammation in TMA. [114-116] Impaired complement regulation leading to a microvascular thrombosis syndrome directly implicates both inflammatory and thrombotic pathways in this form of TMA. In addition to many basic science, animal model, and translational studies, the role of impaired complement regulation in aHUS is supported clinically by the efficacy of plasma exchange in cases in which a soluble complement regulatory factor is defective (e.g., factor H, factor I), and by the general efficacy of the complement inhibiting drug eculizumab. [117-120] The mechanism by which complement activation leads to aHUS is incompletely understood, but the recruitment of inflammatory cells and subsequent EC injury are likely to be key components. [121] There is an emerging concept that the interplay between complement and coagulation is an important factor in all major forms of TMA. [122, 123]

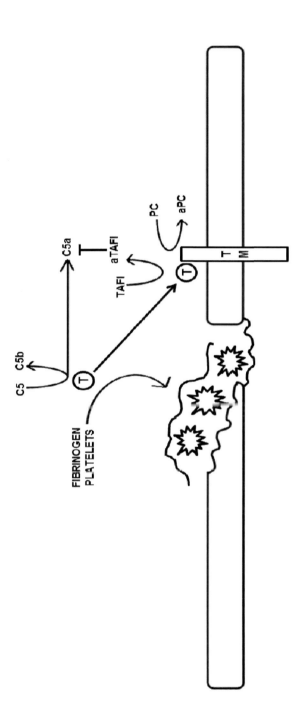

Figure 1. Thrombin (T) plays key roles in both hemostasis and inflammation. Once thrombin binds thrombomodulin (TM), the procoagulant and complement-activating activities are directly inhibited as the thrombin-thrombomodulin complex activates thrombin-activatable fibrinolysis inhibitor (TAFI) and protein C (PC). Activated TAFI (aTAFI) inactivates anaphylatoxins C5a (shown) and C3a (not shown). Activated protein C (aPC) downregulates the coagulation cascade and thrombin production.

The convergence between inflammation and thrombosis has been further established by the discovery that the thrombomodulin-protein C pathway regulates both coagulation and inflammation (Figure 1). Several studies have revealed that thrombomodulin modulates inflammation through both activated protein C-dependent and activated protein C-independent mechanisms. [124] In one study, LPS exposed mice lacking the N-terminal lectin-like domain of thrombomodulin (TM-D1) had reduced survival even though the anticoagulant function of thrombomodulin was intact. [125] This finding confirmed a separate critical function of thrombomodulin in addition to anticoagulation. Another study using TM-D1 mice showed enhanced deposition of C3 and increased severity of inflammatory disease, suggesting a complement regulatory function of thrombomodulin. [126] Subsequent studies showed that thrombomodulin augments factor I-mediated inactivation of C3b as well as thrombin-activatable fibrinolysis inhibitor (TAFI)-mediated inactivation of the anaphylatoxins C5a and C3a. [127-130] The recent discovery of loss of function thrombomodulin mutations in some patients with aHUS confirmed a complement regulatory role of thrombomodulin in this form of TMA. [131-133] Based on these discoveries, recent case reports have demonstrated efficacy of recombinant soluble thrombomodulin in the treatment of aHUS. [134-136]

Conclusion

Accumulating evidence implicates thrombin activation in many if not all forms of TMA. Laboratory and clinical experiences with procoagulant disorders such as sepsis, DIC, and APL suggest the importance of thrombin inhibition in the prevention and treatment of TMA. The role of thrombin regulation and its integral relationship to inflammation is a promising and under-explored area of investigation. Direct thrombin inhibition has shown hints of effectiveness in preventing the onset of HUS in the greyhound model. Alternatively, modulation of the thrombin substrate specificity via soluble thrombomodulin appears to hold promise in the treatment of aHUS. Augmentation of thrombomodulin function by treatment with soluble thrombomodulin or by upregulation by retinoic acid opens a new window of opportunity in the treatment of TMAs. The authors hope this chapter serves to stimulate inquiry into the promising possibility of modulating both inflammation and thrombosis in the treatment of TMAs. Where strategies targeting the downstream procoagulant effects of thrombin may have failed thus far, a strategy targeting upstream regulators of inflammation and thrombosis may succeed.

References

[1]   Radhi M, Carpenter SL. Thrombotic microangiopathies. *ISRN Hematology.* 2012.

[2]   Sadler JE. Von Willebrand factor, ADAMTS13, and thrombotic thrombocytopenic purpura. *Blood.* 2008;112(1):11-8.

[3]   Schwartz J, Winters JL, Padmanabhan A, Balogun RA, Delaney M, Linenberger ML, et al. Guidelines on the Use of Therapeutic Apheresis in Clinical Practice—Evidence-Based Approach from the Writing Committee of the American Society for Apheresis: The Sixth Special Issue. *Journal of clinical apheresis.* 2013;28(3):145-284.

[4]   Sagheer S, Moiz B, Usman M, Khurshid M. Retrospective review of 25 cases of thrombotic thrombocytopenic purpura in Pakistan. *Therapeutic Apheresis and Dialysis.* 2012;16(1):97-103.

[5]   Motto D. Endothelial cells and thrombotic microangiopathy *Seminars in nephrology.* 2012;32(2):208-14.

[6]   van Hinsbergh VW, editor Endothelium—role in regulation of coagulation and inflammation. *Seminars in immunopathology;* 2012: Springer.

[7]   Wu M, KK, Thiagarajan M, P. Role of endothelium in thrombosis and hemostasis. *Annual review of medicine.* 1996;47(1):315-31.

[8]   Kriz N, Rinder CS, Rinder HM. Physiology of hemostasis: with relevance to current and future laboratory testing. *Clinics in laboratory medicine.* 2009;29(2):159-74.

[9]   Saba HI, Saba SR. Vascular Endothelium, Influence on Hemostasis: Past and Present. *Hemostasis and Thrombosis: Practical Guidelines in Clinical Management.* 2014:14.

[10]   Shaz B, Hillyer CD, Abrams C, Roshal M. Transfusion Medicine and Hemostasis: *Blood banking and transfusion medicine: Elsevier Science;* 2013.

[11]   O'Connor SD, Taylor AJ, Williams EC, Winter TC. Coagulation concepts update. *American Journal of Roentgenology.* 2009;193 (6):1656-64.

[12] Mackman N. Role of tissue factor in hemostasis, thrombosis, and vascular development. *Arteriosclerosis, thrombosis, and vascular biology.* 2004;24(6):1015-22.

[13] Brummel KE. Thrombin functions during tissue factor-induced blood coagulation. *Blood.* 2002;100(1):148-52.

[14] Stern D, Nawroth P, Handley D, Kisiel W. An endothelial cell-dependent pathway of coagulation. *Proceedings of the National Academy of Sciences.* 1985;82(8):2523-7.

[15] de Jonge E, Dekkers PE, Creasey AA, Hack CE, Paulson SK, Karim A, et al. Tissue factor pathway inhibitor dose-dependently inhibits coagulation activation without influencing the fibrinolytic and cytokine response during human endotoxemia. *Blood.* 2000;95(4):1124-9.

[16] Mertens G, Cassiman J-J, Van den Berghe H, Vermylen J, David G. Cell surface heparan sulfate proteoglycans from human vascular endothelial cells. Core protein characterization and antithrombin III binding properties. *Journal of Biological Chemistry.* 1992;267 (28):20435-43.

[17] Sadler JE, Lentz SR, Sheehan JP, Tsiang M, Wu Q. Structure-function relationships of the thrombin-thrombomodulin interaction. *Haemostasis.* 1993;23 Suppl 1:183-93.

[18] Esmon CT. The protein C pathway. *CHEST Journal.* 2003;124 (3_suppl):26S-32S.

[19] Van de Wouwer M, Collen D, Conway EM. Thrombomodulin-protein C-EPCR system: integrated to regulate coagulation and inflammation. *Arteriosclerosis, thrombosis, and vascular biology.* 2004;24(8):1374-83.

[20] Schmaier AH, Miller JL. Coagulation and fibrinolysis. In McPherson RA, Pincus MR, editors: *Henry's clinical diagnosis and management by laboratory methods,* ed 22. Philadelphia: Elsevier; 2011. p. 785-800.

[21] Schaller J, Gerber SS. The plasmin–antiplasmin system: structural and functional aspects. *Cellular and Molecular Life Sciences.* 2011;68 (5):785-801.

[22] Brogren H, Karlsson L, Andersson M, Wang L, Erlinge D, Jern S. Platelets synthesize large amounts of active plasminogen activator inhibitor 1. *Blood.* 2004;104(13):3943-8.

[23] Williams EC. Plasma a2-Antiplasmin Activity: Role in the Evaluation and Management of Fibrinolytic States and Other Bleeding Disorders. *Archives of internal medicine.* 1989;149(8):1769-72.

[24] Barthel D, Schindler S, Zipfel PF. Plasminogen is a complement inhibitor. *Journal of Biological Chemistry.* 2012;287(22):18831-42.

[25] Syrovets T, Lunov O, Simmet T. Plasmin as a proinflammatory cell activator. *Journal of leukocyte biology.* 2012;92(3):509-19.

[26] Aird WC. Endothelial cell heterogeneity. *Critical care medicine.* 2003;31(4):S221-S30.

[27] Aird WC. Mechanisms of endothelial cell heterogeneity in health and disease. *Circulation research.* 2006;98(2):159-62.

[28] Aird WC. Phenotypic heterogeneity of the endothelium I. Structure, function, and mechanisms. *Circulation research.* 2007;100(2):158-73.

[29] Aird WC. Phenotypic heterogeneity of the endothelium II. Representative vascular beds. *Circulation research.* 2007;100(2): 174-90.

[30] Bevilacqua M, Pober J, Majeau G, Cotran R, Gimbrone M. Interleukin 1 (IL-1) induces biosynthesis and cell surface expression of procoagulant activity in human vascular endothelial cells. *The Journal of experimental medicine.* 1984;160(2):618-23.

[31] Harker LA. Thrombogenic abnormalities of the endothelium. In: Mc Arthur JR, editor. *Hematology 1992 - Education Program American Society of Hematology.* Anaheim1992.

[32] Bevilacqua MP, Schleef RR, Gimbrone MA, Jr., Loskutoff DJ. Regulation of the fibrinolytic system of cultured human vascular endothelium by interleukin 1. *The Journal of Clinical Investigation.* 1986;78(2):587-91.

[33] Potti A, Ramiah V, Ortel TL. Thrombophilia and Thrombosis in Thrombotic Thrombocytopenic Purpura. *Semin Thromb Hemost.* 2005;31(06):652-8.

[34] Kwaan H. Role of fibrinolysis in thrombotic thrombocytopenic purpura. *Seminars in hematology.* 1987;24(2):101-9.

[35] Kwaan HC. The pathogenesis of thrombotic thrombocytopenic purpura. *Seminars in thrombosis and hemostasis.* 1978;5(3):184-98.

[36] Glas-Greenwalt P, Hall JM, Panke TW, Kant KS, Allen CM, Pollak VE. Fibrinolysis in health and disease: abnormal levels of plasminogen activator, plasminogen activator inhibitor, and protein C in thrombotic thrombocytopenic purpura. *J Lab Clin Med.* 1986;108:415-22.

[37] Kakishita E, Koyama T, Higuchi M, Kunitomi O, Oura Y, Nagai K. Fibrinogenolysis in thrombotic thrombocytopenic purpura. *American journal of hematology.* 1989;32(1):14-9.

[38] Archipoff G, Beretz A, Freyssinet JM, Klein-Soyer C, Brisson C, Cazenave JP. Heterogeneous regulation of constitutive thrombomodulin or inducible tissue-factor activities on the surface of human saphenous-

vein endothelial cells in culture following stimulation by interleukin-1, tumor necrosis factor, thrombin or phorbol ester. *Biochem J.* 1991;273(Pt 3):679-84.

[39]   Conway EM, Rosenberg RD. Tumor necrosis factor suppresses transcription of the thrombomodulin gene in endothelial cells. *Mol Cell Biol.* 1988;8:5588-92.

[40]   Laszik Z, Zhou X, Ferrell G, Silva F, Esmon C. Down-regulation of endothelial expression of endothelial cell protein C receptor and thrombomodulin in coronary atherosclerosis. *American Journal of Pathology.* 2001 159:797-802.

[41]   Lentz SR, Sadler JE. Inhibition of thrombomodulin surface expression and protein C activation by the thrombogenic agent homocysteine. *J Clin Invest.* 1991;88(6):1906-14.

[42]   Lentz SR, Tsiang M, Sadler JE. Regulation of thrombomodulin by tumor necrosis factor-alpha: Comparison of transcriptional and posttranscriptional mechanisms. *Blood.* 1991;77(3):542-50.

[43]   Maruyama I, Okaome T, Sinmyouzu K, al. e. Consumption of endothelial cell-surface thrombomodulin in LPS-induced DIC rats and its improvement by infusion of recombinant thrombomodulin. *Blood.* 1990;76:429a.

[44]   Moore KL, Esmon CT, Esmon NL. Tumor necrosis factor leads to the internalization and degradation of thrombomodulin from the surface of bovine aortic endothelial cells in culture. *Blood.* 1989;73:159-65.

[45]   Scarpati EM, Sadler JE. Regulation of endothelial cell coagulant properties. Modulation of tissue factor, plasminogen activator inhibitors, and thrombomodulin by phorbol 12-myristrate 13-acetate and tumor necrosis factor. *JBiol Chem.* 1996;264(34):20705-13.

[46]   Yu K, Morioka H, Fritze LMS, Beeler DL, Jackman RW, Rosenberg RD. Transcriptional regulation of the thrombomodulin gene. *J Biol Chem.* 1992;267:23237.

[47]   Blann A. Endothelial cell activation, injury, damage and dysfunction: separate entities or mutual terms? *Blood coagulation & fibrinolysis.* 2000;11(7):623-30.

[48]   Haghjooyejavanmard S, Nematbakhsh M. Endothelial function and dysfunction: Clinical significance and assessment. *J Res Med Sci.* 2008;13(4):207-21.

[49]   Thomas L, Good RA. Studies on the generalized Shwartzman reaction I. General observations concerning the phenomenon. *The Journal of experimental medicine.* 1952;96(6):605-24.

[50] Bergstein JM. Glomerular fibrin deposition and removal. *Pediatric Nephrology.* 1990;4(1):78-87.

[51] Moake JL. Haemolytic-uraemic syndrome: basic science. *The Lancet.* 1994;343(8894):393-7.

[52] Zoja C, Buelli S, Morigi M. Shiga toxin-associated hemolytic uremic syndrome: pathophysiology of endothelial dysfunction. *Pediatric Nephrology.* 2010;25(11):2231-40.

[53] Chandler WL, Jelacic S, Boster DR, Ciol MA, Williams GD, Watkins SL, et al. Prothrombotic coagulation abnormalities preceding the hemolytic–uremic syndrome. *New England Journal of Medicine.* 2002;346(1):23-32.

[54] Proulx F, Seidman EG, Karpman D. Pathogenesis of Shiga toxin-associated hemolytic uremic syndrome. *Pediatric research.* 2001;50(2):163-71.

[55] Trachtman H, Austin C, Lewinski M, Stahl RA. Renal and neurological involvement in typical Shiga toxin-associated HUS. *Nature reviews Nephrology.* 2012;8(11):658-69.

[56] Nolasco LH, Turner NA, Bernardo A, Tao Z, Cleary TG, Dong JF, et al. Hemolytic uremic syndrome-associated Shiga toxins promote endothelial-cell secretion and impair ADAMTS13 cleavage of unusually large von Willebrand factor multimers. *Blood.* 2005;106(13):4199-209.

[57] Ray PE, Liu X-H. Pathogenesis of Shiga toxin-induced hemolytic uremic syndrome. *Pediatric Nephrology.* 2001;16(10):823-39.

[58] Grabowski EF, Kushak RI, Liu B, Ingelfinger JR. Shiga toxin downregulates tissue factor pathway inhibitor, modulating an increase in the expression of functional tissue factor on endothelium. *Thrombosis research.* 2013;131(6):521-8.

[59] Bergstein JM, Kuederli U, Bang NU. Plasma inhibitor of glomerular fibrinolysis in the hemolytic-uremic syndrome. *The American journal of medicine.* 1982;73(3):322-7.

[60] Bergstein JM, Riley M, Bang NU. Role of plasminogen-activator inhibitor type 1 in the pathogenesis and outcome of the hemolytic uremic syndrome. *New England Journal of Medicine.* 1992;327 (11):755-9.

[61] Mayer CL, Leibowitz CS, Kurosawa S, Stearns-Kurosawa DJ. Shiga toxins and the pathophysiology of hemolytic uremic syndrome in humans and animals. *Toxins.* 2012;4(11):1261-87.

[62] Coughlin SR. Thrombin signalling and protease-activated receptors. *Nature.* 2000;407(6801):258-64.

[63] O'Brien PJ, Prevost N, Molino M, Hollinger MK, Woolkalis MJ, Woulfe DS, et al. Thrombin responses in human endothelial cells contributions from receptors other than PAR1 include the transactivation of PAR2 by thrombin-cleaved PAR1. *Journal of Biological Chemistry*. 2000;275(18):13502-9.

[64] Minami T, Sugiyama A, Wu S-Q, Abid R, Kodama T, Aird WC. Thrombin and phenotypic modulation of the endothelium. *Arteriosclerosis, thrombosis, and vascular biology*. 2004;24(1):41-53.

[65] Motto D, editor Endothelial cells and thrombotic microangiopathy. *Seminars in nephrology;* 2012: Elsevier.

[66] Motto DG, Chauhan AK, Zhu G, Homeister J, Lamb CB, Desch KC, et al. Shigatoxin triggers thrombotic thrombocytopenic purpura in genetically susceptible ADAMTS13-deficient mice. *Journal of Clinical Investigation*. 2005;115(10):2752-61.

[67] Chauhan AK, Walsh MT, Zhu G, Ginsburg D, Wagner DD, Motto DG. The combined roles of ADAMTS13 and VWF in murine models of TTP, endotoxemia, and thrombosis. *Blood*. 2008;111(7):3452-7.

[68] Hertzke D, Cowan L, Schoning P, Fenwick B. Glomerular ultrastructural lesions of idiopathic cutaneous and renal glomerular vasculopathy of greyhounds. *Veterinary Pathology Online*. 1995;32(5):451-9.

[69] Raife T, Friedman KD, Fenwick B. Lepirudin prevents lethal effects of Shiga toxin in a canine model. Thromb Haemost. 2004;92(2):387-93.

[70] Vitacco M, Avalos JS, Gianantonio CA. Heparin therapy in the hemolytic-uremic syndrome. *The Journal of pediatrics*. 1973;83(2):271-5.

[71] Esmon CT, Owen WG. Identification of an endothelial cell cofactor for thrombin catalyzed activation of protein C. *Proc Natl Aced Sci USA*. 1981;78:2249.

[72] Esmon C, Owen WG. The discovery of thrombomodulin. *Journal of Thrombosis and Haemostasis*. 2003;2:209-13.

[73] Weiler H, Christie P, Beeler DL, Healy AM, Hancock W, Rayburn HB, et al. A targeted point mutation in thrombomodulin generates viable *mice with a prethrombotic state*. Journal of Clinical Investigation 1998;101:1983-91.

[74] Weiler H, Lindner V, Kerlin B, Isermann B, Hendrickson S, Cooley B, et al. Characterization of a mouse model for thrombomodulin deficiency. *Arteriosclerosis, Thrombosis, and Vascular Biology* 2001;21:1531-7.

[75] Healy AM, Rayburn HB, Rosenberg RD, Weiler H. Absence of the blood-clotting regulator thrombomodulin causes embryonic lethality in mice before development of a functional cardiovascular system. *Proc Natl Aced Sci USA.* 1995;92:850.

[76] Esmon C. Protein C anticoagulant system-anti-inflammatory effects. *Seminars in Immunopathology.* 2012;34(1):127-32.

[77] Moore K, Andreoli S, Esmon NL, al. e. Endotoxin enhances tissue factor and suppresses thrombomodulin expression of human vascular endothelium in vitro. *J Clin Invest.* 1987;79:124-30.

[78] Amano K, Tateyama M, Inaba H, Fukutake K, Fujimaki M. Fluctuations in plasma levels of thrombomodulin in patients with DIC. *Thrombosis and Haemostasis.* 1992;68:404-6.

[79] Wada H, Ohiwa M, Kaneko T, Tamaki S, Tanigawa M, Shirakawa S, et al. Plasma thrombomodulin as a marker of vascular disorders in thrombotic thrombocytopenic purpura and disseminated intravascular coagulation. *Am J Hematol.* 1992;39:20-.

[80] Boehme M, Deng Y, Raeth U, Bierhaus A, Zieger R, Stremmel W, et al. Release of thrombomodulin from endothelial cells by concerted action of TNF-a and neutrophils: in vivo and in vitro studies. *Immunology.* 1996;87:134-40.

[81] Kim A, Walinsky P, Kolodgie F, Bian C, Sperry J, Deming C, et al. Early loss of thrombomodulin expression impairs vein graft thromborestinance. *Circulation Research.* 2002;90:205-12.

[82] Cole J, Roberts S, Gallagher M, Giles W, Mitchell B, Steinberg K, et al. Thrombomodulin Ala455Val polymorphism and the risk of cerebral infarction in a biracial population: the stroke prevention in young women study. *BMC Neurology.* 2004;4:21.

[83] Heit J, Petterson T, Owen WG, Burke J, De Anrade M, Melton J. Thrombomodulin gene polymorphisms or haplotypes as potential risk factors for venous thromboembolism: a population-based case-control study. *Journal of Thrombosis and Haemostasis.* 2005;3:710-7.

[84] Festoff B, Ameenuddin S, Santacruz K, Morser J, Suo Z, Arnold P, et al. Neuroprotective effects of recombinant thrombomodulin in controlled contusion spinal cord injury implicates thrombin signaling. *Journal of Neurotrauma.* 2004;21:907-22.

[85] Ikezoe T. Pathogenesis of disseminated intravascular coagulation in patients with acute promyelocytic leukemia, and its treatment using recombinant human soluble thrombomodulin. *Int J Hematol.* 2013.

[86] Kawano N, Kuriyama T, Yoshida S, Yamashita K, Ochiai H, Nakazaki S, et al. Clinical features and treatment outcomes of six patients with disseminated intravascular coagulation resulting from acute promyelocytic leukemia and treated with recombinant human soluble thrombomodulin at a single institution. *Internal medicine.* 2013;52 (1):55-62.

[87] Matsushita T, Watanabe J, Honda G, Mimuro J, Takahashi H, Tsuji H, et al. Thrombomodulin alfa treatment in patients with acute promyelocytic leukemia and disseminated intravascular coagulation: A retrospective analysis of an open-label, multicenter, post-marketing surveillance study cohort. *Thromb Res.* 2014;133(5):772-81.

[88] Warren HS, Suffredini AF, Eichacker PQ, Munford RS. Risks and Benefits of Activated Protein C Treatment for Severe Sepsis. *New England Journal of Medicine.* 2002;347(13):1027-30.

[89] Raife T, Lentz S, Atkinson B, Vesely S, Hessner M. Factor V Leiden: a genetic risk factor for thrombotic microangiopathy in patients with normal von Willebrand factor-cleaving protease activity. *Blood.* 2002;99(2):437-42.

[90] Krieg S, Studt J-D, Sulzer I, Lämmle B, Kremer Hovinga JA. Is factor V Leiden a risk factor for thrombotic microangiopathies without severe ADAMTS13 deficiency? *Thrombosis and Haemostasis.* 2005;94 (12):1186-9.

[91] Fernández G, Te Loo MM, Velden TA, Heuvel LW, Palermo M, Monnens LA. Decrease of thrombomodulin contributes to the procoagulant state of endothelium in hemolytic uremic syndrome. *Pediatric Nephrology.* 2003;18(10):1066-8.

[92] Zeigler ZR, Rosenfeld CS, Andrews DF, Nemunaitis J, Raymond JM, Shadduck RK, et al. Plasma von Willebrand factor antigen (vWF:AG) and thrombomodulin (TM) levels in adult thrombotic thrombocytopenic purpura/hemolytic uremic syndromes (TTP/HUS) and bone marrow transplant-associated thrombotic microangiopathy (BMT-TM). *American Journal of Hematology.* 1996;53(4):213-20.

[93] Castaigne S, Chomienne C, Daniel MT, Ballerini P, Fornaux P, Degos L. All-trans Retinoic Acid as a Differentiating Therapy for Acute Promyelocytic Leukemia. *IClinical Results.* 1990;76:1704.

[94] Koyama T, Hirosawa S, Kawamata N, Tohda S, Aoki N. All-trans retinoic acid upregulates thrombomodulin and downregulates tissue-factor expression in acute promyelocytic leukemia cells: distinct

expression of thrombomodulin and tissue factor in human leukemic cells. *Blood.* 1994;84(9):3001-9.

[95] Falanga A, Iacoviello L, Evangelista V, Belotti D, Consonni R, D'Orazio A, et al. Loss of blast cell procoagulant activity and improvement of hemostatic variables in patients with acute promyelocytic leukemia administered All-*trans*-retinoic Acid. *Blood.* 1995;86(3):1072-81.

[96] Falanga A, Consonni R, Marchetti M, Mielicki WP, Rambaldi A, Lanotte M, et al. Cancer procoagulant in the human promyelocytic cell line NB4 and its modulation by all-trans-retinoic acid. *Leukemia.* 1994;8(1):156-9.

[97] Raife TJ, Demetroulis EM, Lentz SR. Regulation of thrombomodulin expression by All-*trans* Retinoic Acid and tumor necrosis factor-a: Differential responses in keratinocytes and endothelial cells. *Blood.* 1996;88(6):2043-9.

[98] Bulens F, Ibanez-Tallon I, Van Acker P, De Vriese A, Nelles L, Belayew A, et al. Retinoic acid induction of human tissue-type plasminogen activator gene expression via a direct repeat element (DR5) located at -7 kilobases. *Journal of Biolofical Chemistry.* 1995;270(13):7167-75.

[99] Miwa K, Yamada C, Kono T, Osada H. Retinoic acid enhances plasminogen activation on the cell surface. *Thrombosis Research.* 1995;80(1):47-56.

[100] Miyake S, Ohdama S, Tazawa R, Aoki N. Retinoic acid prevents cytokine-induced suppression of thrombomodulin expression on surface of human umbilical vascular endothelial cells in vitro. *Thromb Res.* 1992;68:483.

[101] Ishii H, Horie S, Kizaki K, Kazami M. Retinoic acid counteracts both the downregulation of thrombomodulin and the induction of tissue factor in cultured human endothelial cells exposed to tumor necrosis factor. *Blood.* 1992;80:2556.

[102] Raife TJ, McArthur J, Kisker T, Lentz SR. Remission after 13-cis retinoic acid in a case of refractory thrombotic thrombocytopenic purpura. *Lancet.* 1998;352:454-5.

[103] Görner M, Seggewiss R, Schlenker T, Stremmel W, Ho A. A case of severe refractory thrombotic thrombocytic purpura responding to treatment with 13-CIS retinoic acid. *British journal of haematology.* 2002;117(1):249-50.

[104] Delvaeye M, Conway EM. Coagulation and innate immune responses: can we view them separately? *Blood.* 2009;114(12):2367-74.

[105] Lian ECY, Byrnes JJ, Harkness DR. Two successful pregnancies in a woman with chronic thrombotic thrombocytopenic purpura treated by plasma infusion. *American journal of hematology.* 1984;16(3):287-91.

[106] Scully M, Thomas M, Underwood M, Watson H, Langley K, Camilleri R, et al. Congenital and acquired thrombotic thrombocytopenic purpura and pregnancy: presentation, management and outcome of subsequent pregnancies. *Blood.* 2014.

[107] Denison FC, Roberts KA, Barr SM, Norman JE. Obesity, pregnancy, inflammation, and vascular function. *Reproduction.* 2010;140(3):373-85.

[108] Lupu C, Lupu F, Dennehy U, Kakkar VV, Scully MF. Thrombin induces the redistribution and acute release of tissue factor pathway inhibitor from specific granules within human endothelial cells in culture. *Arteriosclerosis, thrombosis, and vascular biology.* 1995;15 (11):2055-62.

[109] Becker B, Heindl B, Kupatt C, Zahler S. Endothelial function and hemostasis. *Zeitschrift für Kardiologie.* 2000;89(3):160-7.

[110] Hack CE, Zeerleder S. The endothelium in sepsis: source of and a target for inflammation. *Critical care medicine.* 2001;29(7):S21-S7.

[111] Cines DB, Pollak ES, Buck CA, Loscalzo J, Zimmerman GA, McEver RP, et al. Endothelial cells in physiology and in the pathophysiology of vascular disorders. *Blood.* 1998;91(10):3527-61.

[112] Erickson YO, Samia NI, Bedell B, Friedman KD, Atkinson BS, Raife TJ. Elevated procalcitonin and C-reactive protein as potential biomarkers of sepsis in a subpopulation of thrombotic microangiopathy patients. *Journal of clinical apheresis.* 2009;24(4):150-4.

[113] Samia NI, Friedman KD, Gottschall JL, Raife TJ. Hematocrit and C-reactive protein predict treatment response times in ADAMTS13-deficient thrombotic microangiopathy. *Journal of clinical apheresis.* 2011;26(3):138-45.

[114] Loirat C, Frémeaux-Bacchi V. Atypical hemolytic uremic syndrome. *Orphanet J Rare Dis.* 2011;6(1):60.

[115] Roumenina LT, Loirat C, Dragon-Durey M-A, Halbwachs-Mecarelli L, Sautes-Fridman C, Fremeaux-Bacchi V. Alternative complement pathway assessment in patients with atypical HUS. *Journal of immunological methods.* 2011;365(1):8-26.

[116] Kavanagh D, Goodship T. Genetics and complement in atypical HUS. *Pediatric Nephrology.* 2010;25(12):2431-42.

[117] Nürnberger J, Philipp T, Witzke O, Saez AO, Vester U, Baba HA, et al. Eculizumab for atypical hemolytic–uremic syndrome. *New England Journal of Medicine.* 2009;360(5):542-4.

[118] Gruppo RA, Rother RP. Eculizumab for congenital atypical hemolytic–uremic syndrome. *New England Journal of Medicine.* 2009;360(5): 544-6.

[119] Lapeyraque A-L, Malina M, Fremeaux-Bacchi V, Boppel T, Kirschfink M, Oualha M, et al. Eculizumab in severe Shiga-toxin–associated HUS. *New England Journal of Medicine.* 2011;364(26):2561-3.

[120] Loirat C, Garnier A, Sellier-Leclerc A-L, Kwon T. Plasmatherapy in atypical hemolytic uremic syndrome. *Semin Thromb Hemost.* 2010;36(6):673-81.

[121] Noris M, Remuzzi G. Atypical hemolytic–uremic syndrome. *New England Journal of Medicine.* 2009;361(17):1676-87.

[122] Noris M, Mescia F, Remuzzi G. STEC-HUS, atypical HUS and TTP are all diseases of complement activation. *Nature Reviews Nephrology.* 2012;8(11):622-33.

[123] Nayer A, Asif A. Atypical hemolytic-uremic syndrome: the interplay between complements and the coagulation system. *Iranian journal of kidney diseases.* 2013;7(5):340-5.

[124] Ito T, Maruyama I. Thrombomodulin: protectorate God of the vasculature in thrombosis and inflammation. *Journal of Thrombosis and Haemostasis.* 2011;9(s1):168-73.

[125] Conway EM, Van de Wouwer M, Pollefeyt S, Jurk K, Van Aken H, De Vriese A, et al. The lectin-like domain of thrombomodulin confers protection from neutrophil-mediated tissue damage by suppressing adhesion molecule expression via nuclear factor κB and mitogen-activated protein kinase pathways. *The Journal of experimental medicine.* 2002;196(5):565-77.

[126] Van de Wouwer M, Plaisance S, De Vriese A, Waelkens E, Collen D, Persson J, et al. The lectin-like domain of thrombomodulin interferes with complement activation and protects against arthritis. *Journal of Thrombosis and Haemostasis.* 2006;4(8):1813-24.

[127] Van de Wouwer M, Conway EM. Novel functions of thrombomodulin in inflammation. *Critical care medicine.* 2004;32(5):S254-S61.

[128] Bouma BN, Mosnier LO. Thrombin activatable fibrinolysis inhibitor (TAFI) at the interface between coagulation and fibrinolysis. *Pathophysiology of haemostasis and thrombosis.* 2005;33(5-6):375-81.

[129] Campbell WD, Lazoura E, Okada N, Okada H. Inactivation of C3a and C5a octapeptides by carboxypeptidase R and carboxypeptidase N. *Microbiology and immunology.* 2002;46(2):131-4.

[130] Myles T, Nishimura T, Yun TH, Nagashima M, Morser J, Patterson AJ, et al. Thrombin activatable fibrinolysis inhibitor, a potential regulator of vascular inflammation. *Journal of Biological Chemistry.* 2003; 278(51):51059-67.

[131] Campbell W, Okada N, Okada H. Carboxypeptidase R is an inactivator of complement-derived inflammatory peptides and an inhibitor of fibrinolysis. *Immunological reviews.* 2001;180(1):162-7.

[132] Nishimura T, Myles T, Piliposky AM, Kao PN, Berry GJ, Leung LL. Thrombin-activatable procarboxypeptidase B regulates activated complement C5a in vivo. *Blood.* 2007;109(5):1992-7.

[133] Delvaeye M, Noris M, De Vriese A, Esmon CT, Esmon NL, Ferrell G, et al. Thrombomodulin mutations in atypical hemolytic–uremic syndrome. *New England Journal of Medicine.* 2009;361(4):345-57.

[134] Honda T, Ogata S, Mineo E, Nagamori Y, Nakamura S, Bando Y, et al. A novel strategy for hemolytic uremic syndrome: successful treatment with thrombomodulin α. *Pediatrics.* 2013;131(3):e928-e33.

[135] Udagawa T, Motoyoshi Y, Matsumura Y, Takei A, Ariji S, Ito E, et al. Effect of eculizumab and recombinant human soluble thrombomodulin combination therapy in a 7-year-old girl with atypical hemolytic uremic syndrome due to anti-factor H autoantibodies. *CEN Case Reports.* 2014;3(1):110-7.

[136] Kawasaki Y, Suyama K, Ono A, Oikawa T, Ohara S, Suzuki Y, et al. Efficacy of recombinant human soluble thrombomodulin for childhood hemolytic uremic syndrome. *Pediatrics International.* 2013;55(5):e139-e42.

In: Hemolytic Uremic Syndrome   ISBN: 978-1-63463-227-0
Editors: Glenna Clayton   © 2015 Nova Science Publishers, Inc.

Chapter II

Therapeutic Apheresis in Children with Renal Diseases, Especially Hemolytic Uremic Syndrome

Rolf Bambauer[1,] *, Daniel Burgard[2] and Ralf Schiel[3]*
[1]Formerly: Institute for Blood Purification, Homburg, Germany
[2]Heart Center Duisburg, Duisburg
[3]Inselklinik Heringsdorf GmbH, Seeheilbad Heringsdorf, Germany

Abstract

Since the mid 1970s, membrane modules became available, plasma separation techniques have gained in importance in the past few years. The advantages of this method are a complete separation of the corpuscular components from the plasma and due to increased blood flow rate higher efficacy. Furthermore, cell damage – especially to thrombocytes – occurs less using membranes than centrifuges for cell separation [1]. In this time the demand for treatments of children and adolescents was increasing more and more. The problem was to win the

---

* Correspondence address: Rolf Bambauer, MD, PhD. Frankenstrasse 4, 66424 Homburg, Germany. Tel.: 0049/(0)6841/68500. Fax: 0049/(0)6841/68561. E-Mail: rolf.bambauer@t-online.de.

industry to minmize the hollow fibers, the tubes, the extracorporeal blood volume and at last the machine. The use of therapeutic apheresis (TA) in pediatric patients has always been restricted by technical difficulties and the low incidence of diseases requiring this kind of treatment [2]. The development of new, more sophisticated membranes has allowed to new techniques. The adsorption technologies allow the most selective separation of plasma components without the use of substitution solutions.

Based on many years of experience with extracorporeal circulation in end-stage renal disease, the authors try to give an overview of TA in renal diseases. TA has been successfully introduced in a variety of autoantibody-mediated diseases [1]. The updated information on immunology and molecular biology of different renal diseases are discussed in relation to the rationale for apheresis therapy and its place in combination with other modern treatments. The different renal diseases can be treated by various apheresis methods such as therapeutic plasma exchange (TPE) with substitution solution, or with online plasma or blood purification using adsorption columns which contain biological or non biological agents. The following diseases are discussed: hemolytic uremic syndrome (HUS), rapidly progressive glomerulonephritis (RPGN), including anti-glomerular basement membrane antibody glomerulonephritis (anti-GBM RPGN), RPGN with or without glomerular deposition, pauci-immune PPGN, immune complex nephritis (ICN), and various glomerulonephritis with nephrotic syndrome (NS), myoglobulinemic renal failure, acute kidney injury (AKI), and kidney transplant rejection. Pathogenetical aspects are demonstrated in these diseases, in which they are clarified. TA has been shown to effectively remove the auto-antibodies from blood and lead to rapid clinical improvement.

For the renal diseases which can be treated with TA the guidelines of the Apheresis Applications Committee (AAC) of the American Society for Apheresis (ASFA) are cited. The aim of the present review is to describe the solutions adopted to solve technical difficulties related to priming, vascular access and monitoring and then to evaluate clinical results.

Keywords: Therapeutic apheresis, hemolytic uremic syndrome, rapidly progressive glomerulonephritis, anti-basement membrane antibody glomerulonephritis, immune complex nephritis, nephrotic syndrome, myoglobulinemic renal failure, acute kidney injury, kidney transplant rejection

Introduction

TA with hollow fiber moduls is the most used therapy method in nephrology. Nephrologists have an extensive training in the management of blood purification treatments including vascular access, anticoagulation, volume management and prescription for solute clearance [3]. The renal indications for TPE expand the clinical practice of nephrologists. Before the authors discuss the efficacy of TA in renal diseases, several general considerations that may enrich their interpretation of the data deserve mention [4]. There are only a few prospective controlled trials available for TA in children that are of adequate statistical power to allow definitive conclusions to be reached regarding the therapeutic value of plasma exchange. This drawback reflects, in part, the relative rarity of most of the disorders under investigation. To compensate, many investigators have understandably grouped heterogenous diseases together, often retrospectively, and used historical controls. The latter design is potentially hazardous, given that earlier diagnosis, recognition of milder cases, and improved general care over time may be lost as a benefit of plasma exchange. Most histories of many diseases commonly treated by TA (e.g., myeloma cast nephropathy, nephrogenic systemic fibrosis, cryoglobulinemia, systemic lupus erythematosus) are characterized by episodes of exacerbation and remission, further underscoring the importance of adequate concurrent controls [5]:

1. The thresholds for intervention and the details of treatment protocols may vary widely between centers, rendering it difficult to compare studies.
2. TA is primarily used in the treatment of inflammatory renal diseases as an adjunct to conventional immunosuppressive therapy and might be expected a priori to confer only small additional benefit that require large sample size for its detection.
3. Negative studies are inevitably less likely to be published and estimations of efficacy made on the basis of published reports may be based in favour of TA.

For those diseases for which the use of TA is discussed, the guidelines on the use of TA from the Apheresis Applications Committee (AAC) of the American Society for Apheresis (ASFA) are cited [6, 7]. Especially the categorization and indications of different diseases of the AAC are mentioned.

TA includes TPE, immunoadsorption (IA), hemoperfusion (whole blood adsorption), and other adsorption methods. The technical aspects of all these methods are described elsewhere [8]. The most introduced methods are TPE and IA.

This overview is to highlight the disease processes commonly treated with TA in children, and to address the technical considerations pertinent to the provision of safe and effective in pediatric setting. Especially jounger and smaller children will have lower total blood volume and more difficult vascular access. After the Geigy scientific tables from 1970 the total blood volume based on a child´s age weight, ~ 85 mL/kg in normal sized newborns and infants, 80 mL/kg in toddlers and preschool children, 75 – 80 mL/kg in early elementary school children, 70 – 75 mL/kg in older pre-pubertal children, and 70 mL/kg in adolescent [9].

The extracorporeal circuit needs to be primed with a solution that will help maintain intravascular integration such as red cell diluted with saline or 5 % albumin to a hematocrit value near 40 % or a 5 % albumin-electrolyte solution in children who are more stable hemodynamically [10]. Any successful extracorporeal circuit requires adequate vascular access. The vascular access in small children, stiffer and more durable venous catheters are favoured to withstand the negative pressure generated by machine inlet flows, which generally exceed 20 – 40 mL/min. In older children and adolescents with good peripheral extremity vasculature, standard wide-bore 18 – gauge intravenous catheter access can be sufficient [10]. Certain smaller gauge and more flexible catheters are not as optimal for apheresis in children. Anticoagulation therapy can be administered via heparin or anticoagulant citrate dextrose formula A. The most common adverse sequelae of citrate anticoagulation are metabolic alkalosis and hypocalcemia [10]. In these cases calcium infusions are necessary.

Other problems can be multiple psychsocial factors that may play a larger role in performing TA on a child than an adult. In pediatric patients of all ages, undergoing treatments can cause a great deal of anxiety for both the child and any parents or adult caregivers. In these cases taking advantage of clinical staff with prior pediatric experience, or child life specialists are useful [10]. TA in pediatric diseases presents unique challenges and is associated with higher complication rate compared to adults. It is recommended to perform these procedures in specialized centers [11]. In recent years guidelines have been established for implementing TA with regard to the special situation of pediatric patients.

Table 1 shows a compilation from selected literature of most of the pediatric renal diseases that have been treated with TA. In 1988, Bambauer et al. introduced a small system with a small double-head pump (220 x 255 x 95 mm) and a small substitution pump with a special system of tubes for the blood and filtrate line and smaller hemofilter, and very small plasma membrane separators for hemofiltration and TPE treatment for premature infants and newborns [12].

Table 1. Guidelines on the use of TA in clinical practice-evidence based approach [6, 7]

Diseases	Apheresis Applications Committee of ASFA, 2010, 2013		
	TA modality	Category	Recommendation grade
Hemolytic uremic syndrome			
- Complement factor gene mutations	TPE	II	2C
- Factor H antibodies	TPE	I	2C
- MCP mutations	TPE	IV	1C
Rapidly progressive glomerulonephritis			
- RPGN (ANCA associated) Dialysis dependence	TPE	I	1A
- DAH	TPE	I	1C
- Immune complex nephritis dialysis-independence	TPE	IV	2B
Anti-glomerular basement disease (Goodpasture syndrome)			
- Dialysis-dependent, no DAH	TPE	III	2B
- DAH	TPE	I	1C
- Dialysis-independent	TPE	I	1B
Focal segmental glomerulonephritis			
- primary	TPE	III	1C
- secondary	TPE	III	1C
- recurrent (in transplanted kidney)	TPE	I	1B
Renal transplantation, ABO compatible			
- Antibody mediated rejection	TPE	I	1B
- Desensitization, living donor, pos. crossmatch due to donor specific HLA antibody	TPE	I	1B
- Desensitization, high PRA deceased donor	TPE	III	2C
Renal transplantation, ABO incompatible			
- Desensitization, live donor	TPE	I	1B
- Humoral rejection	TPE	II	1B
- Group A2/A2B into B, deceased donor	TPE	IV	1B

Hemolytic-Uremic Syndrome (HUS)

Hemolytic-uremic syndrome is a disease that can lead to acute kidney injury (AKI) and often to other serious sequelae, including death. The disease is characterized by microangiopathic hemolytic anemia, thrombocytopenia and acute kidney injury. The etiology and pathogenesis of HUS are not completely understood, and the therapy of HUS is complicated. After introduction of TA as a supportive therapy in HUS, several authors reported successful treatment using TA in HUS in more than 87 percent of treated patients. The supportive therapy is indicated basically in severe courses of HUS and is superior to available therapy interventions [1]. The pathophysiologic aspects of the different pathogenic types of HUS are discussed by Bambauer et al. [13].

Most cases are associated with infections with entero-hemorrhagic E. coli (EHEC). These bacteria can be transmitted through contaminated food, animal and person to person contact. HUS is one of the most severe complications of a potentially avoidable food-borne infection. Other causes of HUS described as "typical" have to be differentiated since other factors including genetic disorders are of importance. In view of the different courses of HUS, a minimum of three different pathogenetic types which lead to HUS are subdivided. HUS caused by infection, idiopathic HUS (non-Shiga toxin HUS), and HUS in systemic diseases and after toxin exposure [14].

There have been reports of spontaneous recovery from HUS. The total lethality in HUS was first reduced to 20 percent with the introduction of dialysis. If the therapy is administered early enough, two-thirds of cases recover without any impairment. In 10-20 percent of cases, however, lasting renal damage occurs. Other authors reported successful in HUS using TPE [15-17]. In the following years other authors reported successful treatment in HUS using IA with protein-A [18]. Bambauer et al., showed a compilation of therapeutic concepts for HUS implemented up to 2009 that the success of HUS therapy with TPE/HD or IA/HD has been constantly increasing, as numerous reports indicated [13].

The simple plasma infusion after Remuzzi et al. is not sufficient (19). However, substitution of plasma or coagulation factors is often necessary due to the severe coagulation problems in HUS. TA might be more effective than infusions alone, as it removes potentially toxic substances from the circulation. TPE or IA should be considered first-line therapy in situations that limit the amount of plasma that can be infused, such as renal or heart failure. Plasma infusion treatment is contraindicated in S. pneumonia induced non-stx-HUS. It may exacerbate the disease because adult plasma contains antibodies against Thomson-Friedenreich antigen [20].

Michael et al., found in different randomized controlled trials that TPE and/or dialysis as supportive therapy are still the most effective treatments in HUS (21). The outcome was listed for HUS, all-cause mortality, chronic reduced kidney function, and persistent proteinuria or hypertension at last follow up. None of the evaluated interventions such as fresh frozen plasma transfusion or dipyridamole, Shiga toxin binding protein and steroids were superior to supportive therapy alone for any outcomes [21].

The advantage of TA over other therapeutic procedures is that it intervenes at an early stage in the pathogenetic processes by quickly removing immune complexes and toxins. Furthermore, it eliminates fibrinogen, fibrinogen degradation products, and other high molecular complexes, all of which can both support and inhibit coagulation. All other toxins produced by bacteriae and viruses like Shiga-toxin, the pathogenic pathway which follows the activation of the complement system of the factor HF1 with a partial HF1 deficiency and all other toxic substances can be quickly removed by TA.

The rationale for TA in HUS is discussed controversially because of the limited and or conflicting data available in the literature. The rationale is that TA can effectively remove antibody or mutated circulating complements regulators [7]. TA seems a reasonable option considering the poor prognosis of HUS in adults [6]. The role of TA is uncertain but this treatment may be appropriate as supportive therapy under certain circumstances and with a defined therapeutic endpoint because of the high mortality.

In 2010 and 2013 the AAC of the ASFA divided HUS in 3 groups for TPE (Table 1): Group 1 (diarrhea associated HUS) is a HUS due to complement factor gene mutations has the catregory II with the recommendation grade (RG) 2C. Group 2 is a HUS due to autoantibody to factor H (atypical HUS), and has the category I with the RG 2C. Group 3 is the typical HUS <18 years. Group 3 has the category IV with the RG 1C [6, 7]. Due to the various and very different causes, which can lead to a hemolytic-uremic syndrome, there are no exact guidelines available for the therapy of HUS. This will acknowledge that choosing evidence-based therapies are often limited by our incomplete understanding of the various pathogenic cascades. In HUS a supportive therapy is indicated which include control of fluid and electrolyte imbalance, use of dialysis if required, control of hypertension, blood and plasma transfusion as required. Antibiotic treatment of E. coli O157:H7 colitis may stimulate further verotoxin production and thereby increase the risk of HUS. The use of dialysis like hemodialysis or peritoneal dialysis as required daily. However untreated HUS in adults and children may progress to end in organ damage [22]. Platelet transfusion may actually worsen outcome.

TPE or IA is generally performed daily until the platelet count is normal. In the TPE the replacement fluid consists of human albumin-electrolyte solution (5%) in 30 to 70 percent and fresh frozen plasma (FFP) in the remainder. The exchange volume per treatment should be 1–1.5 total plasma volume depending on the severity of the HUS. TPE may reverse the ongoing platelet consumption. By using IA no replacement fluid is necessary only between the treatments FFP or coagulation factors may be transfused if required. An exchange volume of 3–4 L plasma corresponding to whole blood is recommended. The hemodialysis treatment can be combined with the TA.

A large outbreak of diarrhea and the HUS caused by an unusual serotype of Shiga-toxin-producing Escherichia coli (O104:H4) was in Germany in May to July 2011 with 3,167 without HUS and 16 deaths in the patients, and 908 with HUS and 34 deaths [23]. 241 patients with HUS were treated with TPE and 193 patients with TPE and eculizumab. The treatment strategy was dependent on disease severity [24]. TPE and eculizumab in combination seems to be prudent and necessary prior to establishing new treatments guidelines.

Rapidly Progressive Glomerulonephritis (RPGN)

RPGN is a diffuse glomerulonephritis that frequently begins acutely. RPGN is a histologic diagnosis, and can occur from a number of etiologies, including ABM-ab-GN, which is very rare, ANCA, even IgA nephritis (Table 2). Its histological characteristics are usually capillary emboli with necrosis of the capillary walls and semi-lunar formation, and deposition of IgG and C3 along the glomerular basement membrane. Most cases are simultaneously accompanied by acute kidney injury [25]. More than 90 percent of patients with RPGN due to Goodpasture's/anti-GBM RPGN have anti-GBM antibodies in their circulation. The latter are directed against the 28-kd non-colagenous C-terminus of the α3 chain of the type IV collagen, an epitope that is relatively restricted to glomerular and alveolar basement membrane [26]. ANCA GN can be a RPGN, and very few of these patients will also have anti-GBM antibodies. In general, disease activity correlates with the titer of circulating antibodies, and passive transfer experiments have provided compelling evidence that circulating anti-GBM antibodies are nephrotoxic.

The type of lesions in the kidneys depends on the size of immune complexes [27]. If the serum contains a large antigen excess, the complexes are small and therefore pass readily not only through the endothelial layer lining the capillaries in the kidney glomerulus but also across the underlying basement membrane.

Table 2. Immunopathological classification of RPGN (modified after Szczepiorkowski et al. [6, 7])

	RPGN type	Frequency (%)

I	RPGN with linear deposition of IgG due to autoantibodies
	To type IV collagen representing anti-glomerular basement GN (anti-GBM)
	  1. Goodpasture syndrome
	  2. Idiopathic anti-GBM nephritis
	  3. Membranous nephropathy mostly associated with PLA2R antibodies
		15

II	RPGN with granular deposits of immune-complexes
	  1. Post infectious
	    • Post streptococcal GN
	    • Abscesses
	    • Bacterial endocarditis
	  2. Non infectious
	    • Systemic lupus erythematosus
	    • Schönein-Henoch purpura
	    • Cryoglobulinämia
	    • Wegner´s granulomatosus
	    • Polyarteriitis other forms of vasculitis
	    • Solid tumors
	  3. Primary renal diseases
	    • IgG – IgA – nephritis
	    • Membranoproliferative GN
	    • Idiopathic immune – complex nephritis
		24

III	RPGN with or without minimal glomerular deposition (ANCA ab): Pauci-immune glomerulonephritis
	  1. Microscopic vasculitis
	  2. Wegner´s granulomatosus
	  3. Polyarthritis nodosa
		60

The complexes end up outside the blood vessels under the epithelial cells that surround them. The immune complex deposits stimulate the epithelial cells to swell and proliferate. If the serum contains a small antigen excess, the large soluble immune complexes penetrate the endothelial layer but not the basement membrane and are therefore deposited inside the blood vessels under the endothelial cells to swell and proliferate. Simultaneously, the tissue-bound complexes outside and inside the blood vessel activate the complement cascade and through it initiate an inflammatory response that leads to kidney damage to glomerulonephritis [27].

The deposition of circulating immune complexes causes an immune complex nephritis. This results in glomerular immune complex deposits, type IgG. It often occurs after bacterial infections. The frequency of immune complex nephritis is 15 percent [7]. The formation of circulating immune complexes is a physiological process. During the formation of antibodies in the presence of antigens, excessive formation of middle-sized immune complexes occurs. It is possible that genetic disposition plays a large role here. The circulating immune complexes with a molecular weight of approximately 106 Daltons can now, through complementary activation at the basal membranes, lead to respective changes with linear or granular deposits of IgG, IgA, IgE, C3 and to reactive tissue reaction, including necrosis [28].

Other authors found that interleukin-4 (IL-4) has been recently implicated in the pathogenesis of glomerulonephritis. Different others authors presented in vitro the activation by antibodies to proteinase 3 and myeloperoxidase from patients with crescentic glomerulonehritis. They showed that anti-proteinase 3 is more potent in activating neutrophils than in anti-myeloperoxidase in crescentic GN (29). In most cases granular or linear IgG and C3 deposits can be detected in the kidney biopsy by means of the immunofluorescence technique. Granular fluorescence of the glomerular capillary walls indicates a form of immune complex nephritis, while when linear immunoglobulin deposits are presented the term anti-basement membrane antibody glomerulonephritis (Goodpasture syndrome) is used.

After the guidelines on the use of TA in clinical practice-evidence-based approach of the AAC of the ASFA is RPGN not a single disease entity but is a clinical syndrome that can result from a number of etiologies. Histologic classification divides RPGN into three subtypes based on the immunoflourescence pattern on renal biopsy [6, 7] (Table 2):

1) Linear deposition of IgG due to autoantibodies to type IV collagen representing anti-glomerular basement GN (15%).
2) Granular deposits of immune-complexes caused by a variety of GNs including post-streptococcal GN, Henoch Schönlein purpura, IgA nephropathy, membranoproliferative GN, cryoglobulinemia, and lupus nephritis (24%).
3) Minimal immune deposits in the glomerulus with the presence of anti-neutrophil antibodies in the serum. This pauci-immune RPGN also referred to as ANCA-associated RPGN, is seen in Wegner's granulomatosis (WG) and microscopic polyangiitis (MPA) (60%) [6, 7].

The incidence is 0.85 per 100.000/year. Importantly, when discussing RPGN, a number of entities are frequently included in case series and trials, thus confounding results [6]. Therapy consists of administration of high-dose corticosteroid (e.g., methylprednisolone) and cytotoxic immunosuppressive drug (e.g., cyclophosphamide or azathioprine). Other drugs have been used include leflunomide, deoxyspergualin, tumor necrosis factor blockers, calcineurin inhibitors, and antibodies against T cells [6, 7].

The rationale for therapeutic apheresis is that RPGN with dialysis dependence (Cr >6 mg/dL) and RPGN with diffuse alveolar hemorrhage have the Category I with the RG 1A and 1C. RPGN dialysis independent has the Category III with the RG 2C [7] (Table 1). Because of the benefit of TPE in the crescentic GN of anti-GBM, TPE was applied to all causes of RPGN [7]. The role of TPE has been examined in some trials in immune complex GN and in the treatment of pauci-immune GN. Results of other trials indicate that TPE may be beneficial for dialysis-dependent patients presenting with severe renal dysfunction; however is no therapeutic benefit over immunosuppression in milder disease. The predominance of pauci-immune GN cases in these series may account for these results [6]. The frequency of TA is every other day. The volume treated is 1–1.5 total plasma volume, and the substitution solution could be a human-albumin-electrolyte solution. Treatment is for 1–2 week followed by tapering with less frequent treatments. The duration of therapy is not well defined in the literature. Some trials have stopped TA if there is no response after 4 weeks of therapy.

Anti-Basement Membrane
Antibody Glomerulonephritis
(Goodpasture Syndrome, ABM-ab-GN)

In ABM-ab-GN antibodies appear which that are directed against a peptide component of one of the two non-collagen parts of type IV collagen. However, type IV collagen is found not only in the kidney, but also in the vessels of other organs, such as the lung [30]. The mechanisms responsible for the production of antibodies against the antigens are still not clear.

A large number of diseases have been associated with Goodpasture syndrome on the basis of different cases; however, the most consistently reported associations are with membranous nephropathy and anti-neutrophil cytoplasmatic antibodies (ANCA) - associated vasculitis. Only a small part of ANCA GN have anti-GBM ab, mostly its thought to be an environmental or infectious exposure that triggers onset of this diseases. It is reasonible to speculate that for both membranous and ANCA-positive vasculits damage to the kidney elicits an immune response against the GBM, leading to the production of antibodies, which may or may not contribute to disease progression [31]. ANCA GN responds to TPE even when patient on dialysis and anti-GBM GN does not.

The formation of anti-basement membrane antibodies is frequently limited in duration. The autoantibodies cause severe disturbances in the permeability in the lung with significant deterioration in diffusion capacity and hemoptysis. The renal deposition of this autoantibody frequently leads to rapid deterioration in renal functioning, which expresses itself histologically in a necrotizing glomerulonephritis in part. Linear deposits of IgG can be immunohistologically detected both at the basement membrane of the lung, as well as of the kidney [30, 32]. An antigen with a probable size of 26,000–28,000 daltons is considered to be responsible for these deposits, its immunogen epitopes being located on the stable glomerular domain NC1 of collagen IV [32]. The antigen is primarily present in a hexamerous form and forms monomers and dimers [32, 33]. After dissociation, antigen determinants are exposed and can thus bind specific antibodies. This molecule seems to be present in all basal membranes, in particular in those of the glomeruli, renal tubuli, the Bowman capsule, the lung, and the plexus chorioideus, in the placenta, but also in those of the aorta and the small intestine.

The positive effect of TPE on the course of antibody-induced RPGN has been established [34].

In a large study, of 85 patients, Lockwood et al., observed in 1984 that the result of the treatment depended on the extent of kidney damage at the beginning of the therapy. With a serum creatinine of <600 μmol/L (<6.8 mg/dl creatinine) TPE, a significant improvement in renal function was achieved in 15 out of 17 patients (88 percent) [35]. According to an overview by Sieberth et al., in 1983, the single application of an immunosuppressive therapy in patients with Goodpasture syndrome only achieved an improvement in renal function in 18 percent of the cases, while 41 percent of the patients displayed this improvement with a combined therapy of TPE and immunosuppression [36]. With serum creatinin under six mg/dl prior to treatment, the combined therapy achieved a significant improvement in renal function in 66 percent of the cases. Jayne et al., presented in their study a creatinine level lower than 5.8 mg/dl in patients with rapidly progressive glomerulonephritis which will be beneficial with TA [37].

Treatment with TPE also provides the possibility of improvement in cases of pulmonary bleeding, which is based on the same immunological process, even when renal function is already irreversibly impaired. A final long-term prognosis for patients whose condition improved after TPE cannot be made. As basement membrane antibody formation often ceases during treatment, recovery or at least partial recovery is possible.

Despite many new findings, the causes of primary glomerulonephritis are still not fully explained. Therapy cannot in most cases really be purposefully applied, therefore. Thus, the various forms of glomerulonephritis are treated with immunosuppression not only with corticoids, alkylating agents, and cyclosporin A, but also with combinations of almost all of these drugs. Trials with anticoagulants, cyclooxygenase inhibitors, and ACE inhibitors suggest that in addition to an immunological genesis of glomerulonephritis, other factors must also be considered [38]. The combination of corticoids, immunosuppressives, and TPE in varying combinations was the first step in improving the overall prognosis for rapidly progressive glomerulonephritis [38]. In subsequent years, RPGN has been treated with the combination of immunosuppressive drugs and IA with excellent results. But Kaplan reported, that several controlled studies have failed to show a generalized benefit of TPE for all patients with RPGN; however, subset analysis of all these studies showed TPE to be beneficial for patients presenting with severe disease or dialysis dependency [39]. A more recent study of Jayne et al., limited to patients presenting with creatinine levels greater than 5.8 mg/dl [37].

In another study based on TPE trial, de Lind van Wijngaarden et al., observed that chronic and acute tubolointerstitial lesions predict the glomerular filtration rate (GFR) at 12 months, yet is the use of plasma exchange and the number of normal glomeruli on biopsy that remained positive predictors of dialysis independence in the same time interval [40]. This finding is important because it suggests that unaffected glomeruli determine long-term renal outcome at 1 year. In a second study the same group of investigators extended their work in determining the rate of renal recovery [41]. In 69 dialysis-dependent patients who were part of the TPE trial, TPE was superior to pulse methylprednisolone with respect to the change of coming of dialysis. The outcome measure depended on the relative number of normal glomeruli (MEPEX study).

Renal biopsy is very important not only diagnostic, but also has prognostic value in patients with Goodpasture syndrome. When less than 30 percent of the glomeruli underwent crescent formation and the renal function is fairly well-preserved, significant response to therapy and good survival can be expected. In contrast, when more than 70 percent of the glomeruli are crescentic and renal insufficiency is present, the renal disease is often progressive and dialysis and possibly renal transplantation are required. Severe renal failure that causes oliguria reduces the survival rate to 50 percent at 6 months [42].

After the authors opinion, TPE should also be applied in advanced renal insufficiency with oligoanuria, even if, according to Lockwood et al., an improvement in renal function can only be expected in five percent of the cases [1, 35]. In these severe cases TPE treatment and an immunosuppressive therapy should be carried out until no further anti-basement membrane antibodies can be detected in the blood. Immunosuppression should subsequently be continued for a further six months, and with persisting renal insufficiency TPE should be carried out over a further period of six to eight weeks.

Before plasmapheresis was availble to remove autoantibodies, prognosis was poor, and most patients die or were left with permanent renal impairment. In patients with diffuse alveolar hemorrhage (DAH) alone, corticosteroids may effective [42]. Cytotoxic agents like cyclophosphamide or azathioprine, may occasionally reverse the renal failure, but their main function is to control DAH. The current combination therapy of TPE and immunosuppressive drugs is successful if applicated early, i.e., in patients without oliguria who do not require dialysis.

Some oliguric dialysis-dependent patients also show a significant response to this combination therapy, as a result of which dialysis can be discontinued. In contrast, anuric patients do not improve in renal function, and continued dialysis is required; renal transplantation may be considered in these often young patients. Fortunately, the autoimmune process in Goodpasture´s syndrome seems to be limited, as demonstrated by the small number of reported cases of recurrent disease [42, 43].

The authors published in 2013 some results of TA and immune-suppressive therapy in Goodpasture syndrome. According to this set of data, the renal function was positively influenced in 166 out of 302 patients (55 percent), and, additionally, hemoptysis in 45 patients (15 percent). In 107 patients (35.5 percent) the combined therapy consisting of TPE and immunosuppression had no effect either on renal function or on hemoptysis [1]. In addition, the antibody is pathogenic, and the goal treatment is the rapid reduction of those antibodies. Even though there have been only small controlled trials of TPE in the treatment of Goodpasture syndrome, it is now an approved therapy for all patients with rapidly progressive glomerulonephritis and/or pulmonary hemorrhage [44].

To be able to evaluate the final status of TPE in Goodpasture syndrome, however, controlled, randomized prospective studies and comparative studies are necessary. Given that TPE can have a positive effect on this serious condition, however, controlled studies are, for ethical reasons, beyond discussion. Furthermore, there are only approximately six to eight new cases per year for example in Germany; and, up to now, only just over 300-400 patients with Goodpasture syndrome have been registered worldwide (incidence: <1 per 100,000 per year). Such a low number of cases make controlled studies practically impossible.

After the available results and trials, TA is provided a more rapid decrease in anti-GBM antibodies, lower post-treatment serum creatinine level, and decreased incidence of end-stage renal disease (ESRD). Given these results and the integral role of the anti-GBM antibody, TA as a means of rapidly decreasing anti-GBM titers has become the standard of care [39].Other authors showed in their findings highlight the safety, efficacy and feasibility of TPE using membrane filtration [45-47].

A treatment strategy can be:

1) Early initiation of TA is essential to avoid ESRD.
2) Initial prescription is 14 daily 3–4 liters exchange.
3) Continued apheresis may be required if antibody titers remain increased.

4) Steroids, cyclophosphamide, or azathioprine are added to decrease production of anti-GBM antibody and minimize the inflammatory response.

The pulmonary symptoms include breathlessness to overt hemoptysis in Goodpasture syndrome. Chest radiographs are nonspecific. Predisposing factors for anti-GBM included the presence of HLA DRB1*1501 allele, exposure to hydrocarbons, and cigarette smoking [6]. Almost all patients have anti-GBM antibodies detectable in their blood. This is directed towards the α3 type IV collagen, which is found in renal and alveolar basement membrane. In addition, 30 percent of patients will also have detectable ANCA. Patients exhibiting both antibodies behave more like anti-GBM than ANCA-vasculitis in the short-term but more like ANCA-vasculitis in the long-term [6, 7]. In anti-GBM GN, treatment includes the combination of TA, cyclophosphamide, and corticosteroids. In general, the disease does not relapse and therefore patients do not need chronic immunosuppression [7]. The exception is patients with ANCA in addition to anti-GBM antibodies. These patients respond rapidly to treatment, like anti-GBM, but can relapse, like ANCA-associated RPGN. These patients require long-term immunosuppression [6, 7]. The category for TA is I with the RG 1A–1C in anti-GBM disease with dialysis dependence and in DAH [7] (Table 1).

In most patients undergoing TA and immunosuppression, anti-GBM antibodies fall to undetectable levels within 2 weeks and the minimum course of TA should be 14 days. The presence or absence of antibody itself should not be used to initiate or terminate therapy, because antibody is not demonstrable in a small percentage of people with the disease and the antibody may be present in patients without active disease. In those patients with active disease and anti-GBM present, TA should be continues until antibodies fall to undetectable levels [6].

Walsh and the European Vasculitis Study Group (EUVAS) found in 2013 that patients with antineutrophil cytoplasma antibody-associated vasculitis requiring dialysis at diagnosis are at risk for developing and ESRD or dying [48]. Short-term results of a trial comparing TPE to intravenous methylprednisolone suggested TPE improved renal recovery. But after Walsh and the EUVAS the long-term follow-up of patients with severe ANCA-associated vasculitis comparing TPE to intravenous methylprednisolone treatment is unclear. Further research is required to determine the role of TPE in this disease.

Immune Complex Nephritis (ICN)

Many types of glomerulonephritis are initiated by the deposition of immune complexes, which induce tissue injury via either engagement of Fc receptors on effector cells or via complement activation [49]. The generation of antibody and subsequent tissue deposition of immune complexes (IC) is thought to trigger the pathogenic consequences of systemic autoimmune disease. Modulation of the autoantibody response disrupts pathogenesis by preventing the formation of ICs; however, uncoupling IC formation from subsequent inflammatory response seems unlikely because of the apparent complexity of the IC-triggered inflammatory cascade [50]. In idiopathic symptomatic RPGN, which is frequently caused by an immune complex nephritis, the therapeutic concept is not as clear-cut as with anti-glomerular basement membrane antibody nephritis. Sieberth et al., demonstrated in a study that a combined therapy of TPE and immunosuppression is superior to immunosuppressive therapy alone [51]. They also found that an improvement in renal function is possible in more than 60 percent of cases, if either pulse therapy (high dose therapy with corticosteroids) or TPE is administered. They therefore propose to first implement the pulse therapy and, if unsuccessful, to then apply TPE. Matic et al., reported their results with the treatment of immunoadsorption (IA) based on specific binding to either staphyloccoccal protein protein-A or sheep polyclonal antibodies directed against human IgG [52]. In 26 patients with different types of immune complex nephritis, 602 IA sessions were performed. Between 60 and 80 percent of IgG was eliminated, depending on the treated plasma. In view of the devastating pathophysiologic consequences of interaction between circulation immune complexes and the basement membrane, the authors share the opinions of Lockwood et al., that TPE in combination with immuno-suppression should be carried out as quickly as possible [35]. The authors published a compilation of some published therapeutic results from different authors. Not included was RPGN resulting from diseases such as systemic lupus erythematosus, Schonlein-Henoch purpura, cryoglobulinemia, Wegener's granulomatosis, or vasculitis [1]. In almost 64 percent of the cases, an improvement or recovery was achieved with the combined TPE and immunosuppression therapy. It is decisive to commence the therapy at as early a stage as possible, while renal function is not yet seriously impaired. Pusey et al., recommended TPE for severe cases of immune complex nephritis [53].

RPGN with or without Glomerular Deposition (ANCA ab) Pauci–Immune RPGN

Approximately 60 percent of patients with RPGN present with crescentic glomerulonephritis characterized by few or absent immune deposits, the so-called pauci-immune RPGN. Patients with this disease have either Wegner's granulomatosis, ANCA-ab associated vasculitis, polyarthritis nodosa, or "renal-limited" pauci-immune GN (Table 2).

These diagnoses may represent a spectrum of manifestations of a single disease, because there is marked overlap of clinical and histopathologic features, and several patients have anti-neutrophil cytoplasmatic antibodies in their blood which are more common that anti-GBM. The concentration of circulating ANCA correlate with the disease activity in some patients, and ANCA may contribute to the pathophysiology of pauci-immune RPGN through reactivity with neutrophils or endothelial cells, and other inflammatory mechanisms [30, 54].

The prognosis of pauci-immune RPGN in general has been poor. Precise therapy therapeutic recommendations are difficult to obtain from the literature, because most series comprise patients with different types of RPGN. However, available data suggest that 80 percent of such patients progress to ESRD without therapy with high dose immunosuppression or cytotoxic drugs [29]. Some trials have evaluated the efficacy of TA as an adjunct to conventional immunosuppressive in patients with pauci- immune RPGN [39, 55, 56].

The results of the randomized trials argue against a role for TA in milder forms of pauci–immune RPGN, but suggest a potential benefit when TA is used as an adjunct to conventional immunosuppressive therapy in patients with severe disease. This relative lack of efficacy probably reflects the efficiency of conventional immunosuppressive agents in halting inflammation and preserving renal function in most patients. These conclusions are supported by the results of uncontrolled trials, suggesting a response rate of 70 percent in patients with RPGN treated with TA, similar to that of patients treated with immunosuppressive therapy with a response rate of 60 percent. In most cases of RPGN, a treatment of TA in the early phase of the disease seems to be necessary.

Hasegawa et al. reported successful treatment using a combinatination of cytapheresis and standard immuno-suppressive therapy of prednisolone and cyclophosmide. In five patients with a myeloperoxidase antineutrophil cytoplasmatic antibody associated vasculitis, the renal function improved and the pulmonary hemorrhage disappeared [54]. Other authors reported of successful treatments with immunoadsorption and immunosuppressive therapy [56, 57].

In the above mentioned MEPEX study, de Lind van Wingaarden et al., showed that in patients with dialysis-dependent, ANCA-associated vasculitis, the chances of recovery differ depending on the type of adjunctive treatment, the percentage of normal glomeruli and glomerulosclerosis, the extent of tubular atrophy, and the presence of arteriosclerosis. Even with an ominous biopsy at diagnosis in combination with dialysis dependence, the chance of renal recovery exceeds the chance of therapy-related death when the patient is treated with plasma exchange as adjunctive therapy [41]. But more further studies are necessary.

Therapy Recommendations for RPGN

RPGN therapy possibilities were extended in recent years to include TA. Antigens, antigen-antibody complexes, and immune complexes can be eliminated from the blood with the aid of plasma exchange. A corresponding therapy enables immunomodulation through suppression or stimulation of antibody formation, as well as a temporary remission of the inflammation through inhibition of the mediators. A combined TA and immunosuppression therapy seems to us to be advisable, particularly in view of the unfavorable prognosis for RPGN, with its complex causes.

The following therapy recommendation is based on the few uncontrolled and controlled studies available [29, 37, 39, 51, 58-60]. TA is indicated in combination with an immunosuppressive therapy with prednisolone (intravenous pulse therapy, or oral therapy), cyclophosphamide (intravenous pulse therapy or oral therapy), or azathioprine in the following cases:

1) RPGN with serum creatinine under 5.8 mg/dl without oliguria in anti-GBM disease.
2) All severe forms of RPGN with or without ANCA ab, like the pauci-immune complexes, (Cr >6 or patient on dialysis).
3) Goodpasture syndrome with life-threatening hemoptysis, or diffuse alveolar hemorrhage from ANCA or MPA independent of renal function status.

4) Preparation for kidney transplant with anti-basement membrane antibodies still detectable in the serum.

Although Lockwood et al. found that an improvement in renal function only occurred in five percent of the patients with RPGN and oligo-anuria and a serum creatinin of <600 μmol/l, despite possible side-effects, it is advisable, to commence plasmapheresis treatment as soon as possible to achieve an improvement [35]. A more recent study limited to patients presenting with creatinine levels greater than 5.8 mg/dl (>512 μmol/l) appears to support this conclusion. Madore et al., recommended to treating all severe forms of RPGN with or without ANCA antibodies with a combination therapy of conventional immunosuppressive therapy and TA [4]. The authors recommend at least four plasma exchange sessions during the first week of immunosuppressive therapy, using four liter exchanges and albumin-electrolyte solution as replacement fluid. With high titers of circulating immune complexes or other antibodies, which could damage the kidney and other organs, IA with protein-A or sheep polyclonal antibodies can be more effective than the TPE procedure. Table 1 summarizes the guidelines on the use of TA in RPGN [6, 7].

In summary, TA used for renal indications, even in elderly patients is relatively safe. Trends towards death in elderly patients may be multi-factoriel and not necessary related to TA [61]. TA may be decrease end point of end-stage renal disease or death in patients with RPGN. TA in combination with immunosuppressive therapies including biologics seems to be more effective as TA alone, but additional trials are required.

Glomerulonephritis with Nephrotic Syndrome (NS)

Classification is classified morphologically, and thus does not provide a uniform description of the disease. Differing etiologies can result in considerable variations in the clinical features, as well as course and prognosis. Consequently, it is difficult to establish generally applicable therapeutic concepts and customized treatment for the individual patient is the norm. The variable clinical courses of this heterogenous disease group render it almost impossible to carry out controlled therapy studies. Both clinical successes and failures are to be found, as are therapy-produced complications, e.g., infections, sterility, loss of hair, and others [62]. The benefits of immunosuppressive therapy must be weighed against these complications. As the aim of therapy for glomerulonephritis is to prevent terminal renal insufficiency and the risks of nephrotic syndrome, some therapeutic possibilities are discussed here.

It is postulated that the cause of nephrotic syndrome lies in changes in the electrophysiological characteristics of the filtration barriers and of the plasma proteins. The anionic charge on albumin is retained by the negative charge of the glomerular filter - including the basement membrane and the epithelium - obviously play a decisive role. Hemodynamic changes, such as increase in venous pressure, can favour the filtration of proteins. Strutz et al., drew attention to an impressive correlation between the degree of proteinuria and the level of the LDL/HDL quotients, as a means of measuring the atherogenic risk [63].

Nephrotic syndrome of various GN often reacts to corticosteroids in varying doses, administered over a period of 4-8 weeks. Patients with frequent relapses are also treated with 2-3 mg/kg BW/day cyclophosphamide [64]. Cyclosporin A has also been successfully applied in nephrotic syndrome. Palla et al., reported on high doses of immunoglobulin (IgG) for nephrotic syndrome. They administered 0.4 g/kg BW IgG on three successive days and repeated this every 21 days over a period of one year [65]. Other therapeutic measures for nephrotic syndrome are anticoagulants, thrombocyte inhibitors, ACE inhibitors, immunosuppressive drugs, lipid reducers, biologics, and diets [66-68].

The prognosis for *focal sclerosing glomerulosclerosis* (FSGS), which is usually accompanied by nephrotic syndrome, is considerably less favorable. Cases with nephrotic syndrome are recorded as having a survival rate of 70 percent after six years. Without nephrotic syndrome, this rate reaches 85 percent. Patients with this form of glomerulonephritis are comprised of steriod–sensitive and a steroid-non-sensitive groups, and a appropriate therapy must be selected. Non-reaction to steroids is an indication for a trial therapy with cyclophosphamide, chlorambucil, or cyclosporin or other immunosuppressive therapy [69, 70]. FSGS is caused by a variety of factors, however, one type that recurs after transplantation and has been associated with circulating factors, can be treated with TA.

Briggs et al., previously reported in 1998 the use of mycophenolate mofetil in 7 partients, whom a substantial improvement in proteinuria was observed [71]. Cattran et al., performed in 2004 an open-label, 6 months trial of mycophenolate mofetil in 18 patients with biopsy-proven FSGS who was resistent to corticosteroid therapy. Seventy-five percent had also failed to respond to a cytotoxic agent and/or cyclosporine A. An improvement in proteinuria was seen in 44 percent of the patients after 6 months. However, no patient achieved a complete remission. In addition, relapses were common after therapy was discontinued [72]. Other therapies have been used in patients with FSGS who prove resistant to standard treatment. Partial remission has been observed in a few case reports using tacrolimus [73].

In the case of resistance to medication or severe progression of the disease, additional TA therapy should be considered, as a continuing treatment given once a week, or every two weeks, or once a month. After transplantation, as many as 40 percent of patients with nephrotic syndrome have recurrences. The glomerular abnormalities in patients with established disease include focal and segmental glomerulosclerosis and hyalinosis, although fusion of epithelial-cell foot processes may be the only abnormality early in the course of disease [74, 75]. It has been proposed that because some patients with recurrent focal glomerulosclerosis have a response to treatment with plasma exchange, LDL apheresis and IA there may be different circulating factors that alter the glomerular barrier to protein filtration [76, 77].

In six patients with focal sclerosing glomerulonephritis, whose renal insufficiency increased despite immunosuppressive therapy, an additional plasma exchange treatment was carried out. Three patients already showed rapid improvement after six or seven sessions of TPE treatment, both with regard to proteinuria and renal insufficiency. The other three patients with acute nephrotic syndrome and protein loss of 20–35 grams in 24 hrs were, after an intensive initial exchange phase, given chronic TPE treatment for 2-4 months, depending on the symptoms. One patient died in the postoperative phase after a stomach operation. All patients were additionally treated with cyclosporin A in a dosage of 2.5-3.5 mg/kg BW/day. In four out of the patients terminal renal insufficiency has been prevented through the administration of additional TPE treatment over a period of 16-20 months [1].

Dantal et al., reported that adsorption of plasma protein decrease urinary protein excretion in patients with recurrence of the NS after renal transplantation [78]. They postulated that the presence of immune complexes in which the factors conductive to albuminuria were active only when they were dissociated from immunoglobulin. They also noted, and that the possibility that the factors could be attached to immunoglobulin through binding to the constant heavy-chain part of the molecule. Pusey et al., recommended in patients with FSGN TPE as a rapid onset of proteinuria following renal transplantation [53].

In the guidelines on the use of TA from the AAC of the ASFA has the primary and secondary FSGS the Category III with the RG 1C, and for the FSGS recurrent the category I with the RG 1B [6, 7] (Table 1). After the guidelines FSGS is a histologically characteristic finding in renal biopsies characterized by focal areas of sclerosis of some glomeruli adjacent to other intact glomeruli. Several FSGS histological variants (cellular, collapsing, tip lesion, perihilar, and not otherwise specified) have been described [7]. FSGS can be primary or secondary to a variety of entities such as obesity, reflux nephropathy, HIV infections, and heroin use. Since at least 50 percent of patients with FSGS progress to renal failure within 5 years, many undergo renal transplants. Unfortunately, about 20 percent of patient will experience a recurence in the renal allograft, especially in children. Recurrent disease is diagnosed by new onset of proteinuria, which should be aggressively treated to slow or arrest progression to renal insufficiency and graft loss. Patients who lost grafts due to recurrent FSGS have >80 percent chance of developing the same lesion in subsequently transplanted kidneys [7].

The treatment in native kidneys with FSGS is primarily with corticosteroids for at least 6 months prior to trying second-line agents such as cyclophosphamide, chlorambucil, or azathioprine. For resistant cases TPE is being currently an option. On the other hand several investigators worldwide have used TPE in the management of patients with FSGS in transplanted organs, in an attempt to save the graft. Although there is no standardized treatment for recurrent FSGS posttransplant, the majority of regimens use a combination of an immune-suppressant such as cyclophosphamide, biologics, and TPE. Other therapeutic options include high-dose cyclosporine, angiogenesis converting enzyme inhibitors, and indomethacin and/or tacrolimus. Another approach to prevent recurrent FSGS is several sessions of pre-emptive TPE immediately prior to and following the transplant [6]. More recently, rituximab and mycophenolate mofetil have also been used in conjunction with diagnosed in order to halt the process and maintain renal function [6, 7].

In only certain FSGS patients appears to contain an ill-defined "permeability factor", probably a glycoprotein of molecular weight of 30–50 kDa that includes profound leakage of albumin when incubated with isolated rat glomeruli. Such factor is removed by TPE and the decrease in serum concentration coincides with improvement in proteinuria. Since it is thought that the immediate onset of proteinuria following transplant is mediated by this factor, prophylactic TPE may be instituted in high risk patients. A few reports describe the use of Staphylococcal protein-A columns in recurrent FSGS. The duration of the procedure is to begin with three daily exchanges followed by at least six more TPE in the subsequent 2 weeks, for minimum of nine procedures. Tapering should be decided on a case by case basis and is guided by the degree of proteinuria. Timing of clinical response is quite variable and control of proteinuria may take several weeks to months. Some patients have received long-term monthly exchanges as maintenance therapy [6, 7]. The treated volume is 1–1.5 total plasma volume. The replacement fluid is an electrolyte-albumin solution, and the frequency daily or every other day.

The nephrotic syndrome consisting of massive proteinuria, hypoalbuminemia, edema, and hyperlipidemia, is a common complication of glomerular disease in children and adults. The annual incidence of nephrotic syndrome ranges from 2–7 per 100,000 children, and prevalance from 12–16 per 100,000. There is epidemiological evidence of a higher incidence of NS in children aged below 10 years from South ASIA [67]. The primary cause of NS is idiopathic [75].

There is evidence pointing to a role of the immune system in *pediatric minimal change glomerulonephritis (MCGN)*. Another hypothesis has described an association between allergyand MCGN in children. Relapses in this of syndrome are triggered commonly by minor infections and occasionally by reactions to be stings or poisoning. Abnormalities of both humoral and cellular immunity have been described. Finally, the induction of remissions by corticosteroid, alkylating agents, or cyclosporine therapy provides indirect evidence for an immune etiology. None of these observations, however, provides direct evidence of immunologically mediated pathogenesis [79].

Although they are massively proteinuric, patients with MCGN, do not have a generalized glomerular leak to macromolecules. The clearance of neutral macromolecules in MCGN is actually less than normal over a range of molecular radii. In contrast, the clearance of anionic macromolecules is significantly increased. This and several other lines of evidence suggest that proteinuria results from a loss of fixed negative charges of anionic glycosaminoglycans in the glomerular capillary wall [80]. The mechanisms through which these charges are lost are unknown. There are different hypotheses. The traditional view is that massive albuminuria, in NS causes a decrease in intravascular oncotic pressure, which allows extravasation of fluid and hypovolemia, increased aldosterone and antidiuretic hormone secretion, and renal salt and water retention. An alternative explanation for retention of salt and water in NS is a decreased glomerular filtration rate, with a decreased filtration fraction [79].

Minimal change glomerulonephritis usually takes a benign course and can be well treated with customary therapy measures. In severe cases, therapy with prednisolone and cyclophosphamide over a period of 8 to 12 weeks is indicated [81, 82]. Cyclosporin has shown some efficacy in steroid-resistant NS (65). Musco et al., reported significantly rapid faster relief from steroid–resistant NS by using LDL apheresis than from steroid monotherapy [83].They showed that a rapid improvement of hypercholesterolemia by LDL apheresis in steroid–resistant NS will provides more rapid relief from NS than from steroid therapy alone. Other authors recommended in steroid-resistant NS intravenous steroids in high dose with alkylating agents, cyclophosphamide oral or pulse cyclophosphamide and mycophenolate mofetil [65, 84, 85].

Membranoproliferative glomerulonephritis (MPGN) usually occurs in combination with nephrotic syndrome and hypertension. The occurrence of nephrotic syndrome signifies a poorer prognosis. The effectiveness of medication with corticosteroids, cyclophosphamides, anticoagulants, and intravenous immunoglobulins has not yet been established. This is also true for pulse therapy [85]. Experience with TA, especially with protein-A immunoadsorption has been presented by Esnault et al., and Dantal et al. They reported of successful treatment with protein-A IA in patients with relapsing nephrotic syndrome [86, 87]. MPGN from cyoglobulinemia could be an indication for TA, too.

The symptoms displayed in mesangioproliferative glomerulonephritis are not usually homogeneous. The prognosis is poorer if the condition is accompanied by nephrotic syndromeand hypertension. Here also, there are varying opinions exist with regard to corticosteroid and cytostatic therapy. Nephrotic syndrome justifies a trial therapy with cyclophosphamide. In view of the uncertainty in drug therapy in this form of glomerulonephritis, three patients were treated additionally with TPE. In the case of two patients, only a few treatment sessions were required in order to normalize renal function, although one patient had to be temporarily hemodialysed due to acute kidney injury. The third patient with accompanying acute nephrotic syndrome (proteinuria 20-25 g/24 hrs.) received TPE treatment regularly over a period of two years. Nevertheless terminal renal insufficiency occurred, which finally made chronic hemodialysis necessary [1]. Although, TA is indicated in severe cases of various types of glomerulonephritis. In severe, drug therapy-resistent cases, a combined TA and immunosuppression therapy is recommended, regardless of the degree of renal insufficiency [76].

Acute nephrotic syndrome in particular seems to be favourably influenced by regular TA treatment, for on the one hand dysproteinemia and thus the edema can be improved and, on the other hand, human albumin can be administered in larger doses. TA is theorectically a way of achieving an improved effect on the basal membrane. The elimination of cholesterol, LDL, and triglycerides might also reduce the atherogenic risk for these patients and thus also prevent progression. TA should be considered as a useful therapeutic tool in the management of this disease [77]. The reports of the therapy of NS with more selective TA procedures like cascade filtration, IA, and LDL apheresis are very encouraging and show a possibility for treating severe cases of NS, if drug therapy fails [86-89]. As in the case of other renal diseases, controlled prospective studies are needed.

Myoglobulinemic Renal Failure

An acute myolysis can induce severe disturbances of the renal function. Free myoglobin with a molecular weight of 17,800 Dalton can be eliminated rapidly by a normal functioning kidney. Massive increase of myoglobin and their derivates in the blood as in acute crushing injuries and mass trauma is highly nephrotoxicity and causes a decreased circulation in the kidney and/and a metabolic acidosis. Acute kidney injury can develop rapidly [90]. Observations showed that, by along with myoglobin, peroxide free radicals of can be released. These can induce a dissiminated intravascular coagulation (DIC), and can damage thrombocytes, the endothelium of the vessels, and disturb the metabolism of prostglandine synthesis.

Rhabdomyolysis is also a clinical syndrome in which the contents of injured muscle cells leak into the circulation. This leakage results in electrolyte abnormalities, acidosis, clotting disorders, hypovolemia, and acute kidney injury. A lot of conditions, both traumatic and non-traumatic, can lead to rhabdomyolysis. Intervention consists of early detection, treatment of the underlying cause, volume replacement, urinary alkalinization, and aggressive diuresis or hemolysis. Patients with rhabdomyolysis often require intensive care [91].

Elimination of myoglobin from plasma may be enhanced by TPE in patients with acute kidney injury [92]. Endothelin, a vasoconstrictive peptide which includes 21 aminoacids, has a strong vasoconstrictive effect in the glomeruli. It leads to hypoxia and hypotension of the endothelium which causes the endothelium to an increased release of endothelin. Siebenlist et al., reported that in three patients with severe myoglobulinemia sufficient to cause renal failure, hemodialysis treatment could be prevented when TPE was used in an early stage [93].

The effect of TPE in the case of three patients with myolysis was very impressive. After operative removal of an abdominal glioblastoma, a one-year-old girl with myoglobulinemic muscular dystrophy and acute kidney injury displayed rapid normalisation of renal function, after three TPE and four HD treatment sessions [1]. Similar normalization in renal functioning was observed in the case of a 77-year-old patient with myoglobulinemic AKI after one TPE session with three liters. Also in another case, a 19-year-old female patient, who suffered from malignant hyperthermia and AKI after administration of an anaesthetic during tonsillectomy, was cured after three sessions of plasmapheresis. In particular in the case of malignant hyperthermia, which is rare but reaches a mortality rate of 60–70 percent, TPE seems to improve the poor prognosis, if applied at an early stage [1].

Yang et al., used TPE in a case of rhabdomyolysis complicated with increased serum bezafibrat level. They advocated that bezafibrate being highly protein bound is unlikely to be cleared by hemodialysis. TPE was safe and effective in addition to supportive care for rhabdomyolysis associated with bezafibrate [94]. Ronco reported that attempts to use TPE in myoglobulinemia have resulted in higher sieving coefficients, but notes limitations due to low volume exchanges [95]. Swaroop et al., described a case of an 82-years old male patient who developed rhabdomyolysis while taking a combination of simvastatin and gemfibrozil and was successfully treated with TPE [96]. Improvement in kidney function when it does occur does so slowly over months of supportive care and dialysis. But there are only a few cases of rhabdomyolysis reported in literature. Most are case reports. Other authors showed that neither plasmapheresis nor hemodiafiltration has been successful in patients with myoglobulinemic renal failure. Fortunately most patients eventually regain normal kidney function [97]. In the case of myoglobulinemic renal failure: TPE interrupts, stops, or eliminates:

1) the toxic effects of myoglobulin and its derivates,
2) the occurrence of disseminated intravascular coagulation through released tissue thromboplastin,
3) non-physiological synthesis of coagulation factors in the liver, the sequestration of active coagulation factors, and metabolic products from the affected tissue.

Acute Kidney Injury (AKI)

The renal diseases are expanded with some notes of acute kidney injury as an independent disease [98]. The variety of the causes that can trigger AKI justifies a close examination of this disease. Acute renal insufficiency means reversible renal damage with oligo-anuria. AKI presents unique, life threatening and organ threatening therapeutics challenges that require prompt accurate diagnosis and treatment. In rare cases, AKI can also take a polyuric course. Damage to the kidneys varies depending on the degree and duration of pre-renal, renal or post-renal disorders (noxae). It is reversible only after the elimination of the noxae; in the case of structural disorders only after its repair; or it can remain irreversible. AKI is also defined as an acute over hours or days developing renal function damage, which is measured by the glomerular filtration rate (GFR). Other renal functions are changed and decreased in AKI, such as the excretion of metabolic products and drugs, the reabsorption of filtrated substances, the regulation in acid-base and electrolyte disorders, and different endocrinological functions. The incidence of AKI is 2–5 percent in inpatients and up to 10-30 percent with intensive medical. The mortality has essentially remained unchanged in the last four decades and at 30 to 80 percent is very high. Although in the last years considerable progress has been made in the dialysis technology and intensive medical care therapy. AKI is the most frequent and expensive renal disease with the highest course of morbidity and mortality in hospitals [99].

As the causative noxae of AKI must be eliminated at the time of insult to the kidney and before it has completely destroyed, they can be influenced primarily during the period in which they act on the kidney. Thereafter, further measures against the noxae are no longer effective; all that then remains is life-long dialysis and/or kidney transplantation [99]. Given the new treatment possibilities, the customary classification of these factors in pre-renal, post-renal, and renal disorders is simplistic from a therapeutic point of view [98].

1) A reduction in renal blood supply that is, having quantitative effect: this group comprises blood flow disorders or noxae. It covers only a part of the pre-renal disorders as commonly classified: circulatory-ischemic disorders such as reduced blood pressure or volume, which can be directly influenced therapeutically, if at all.

2) A qualitative change in renal blood supply: this group includes endogenous or exogenous substances that circulate in the blood and

have a damaging effect on kidney tissue. This group comprises plasma disorders or noxae and includes all endogenous and exogenous toxins, metabolic, and decomposition products, as well as immunologically active substances that circulate in the blood and can damage the kidneys [100]. Many of these plasma disorders can be influenced by therapeutic apheresis. This justifies classification of these pathogenetic factors of an acute kidney injury in a group of their own.

3) Postrenal disorders and damage to the parenchyma of the kidney via obstruction: this is the group urination disorders or noxae. It comprises postrenal disorders, with the exception of intratubular obstruction through substances originally circulating in the blood that precipitate in the tubule lumen (urates, hemoglobin, myoglobin) as a result of urine concentration. Therapy varies according to the nature of the postrenal disorder and is usually treated by urologists [98].

With regard to the treatment of plasma disorders in particular, plasmapheresis opens up a new approach. Conventional therapeutical methods are to be applied to blood flow and postrenal disorders. Of course, in AKI it is important to eliminate or to influence all factors which can lead to AKI and to ensure sufficient administration of parenteral calories, including amino acids, glucose, and fatty solutions [99]. There are no guidelines available for the therapy of AKI. In specially severe or therapy resistant course of AKI the following TA methods could be discussed and implemented:

1) Conventional plasma exchange with hollow fibers could be implemented alone or in combination with dialysis treatments, and 1–5 treatments are recommended every 1–2 days depending on the course and severity of the AKI (98).

2) Selective plasma separation, such as cascade filtration, biological or non-biological adsorption methods, and whole blood adsorption are available. One to maximum of 3 treatments are recommended with an exchange volume of 3 to 4 L plasma corresponding to whole blood.

Up to now, there have not been enough controlled studies of TA used in the treatment of AKI: therefore the physician who treats patients with AKI must decide for himself, wether the introduction of TA in AKI is indicated or not. It is useful to discuss the risk factors and therapeutic modalities with all persons involved in such cases.

Despite the intensive and costly therapeutic modalities in AKI, the mortality of the AKI is always high, at 30–80 percent, and this has not essentially changed in the last four decades [99]. Approximately twice as many patients with severe diseases, such as multi-organ failure and AKI, die in intensive care units when compared with patients without AKI. These patients die not as a result of AKI, but because of the different complications that follow AKI.

Considering these facts and the inevitable unfavorable prognosis of the AKI, it is possible to add the option of therapeutic apheresis to the conservative and extracorporeal therapies [74]. More of controlled studies should be done to improve the clinical outcome and decrease the high costs of this therapeutic method.

Early implementation of TA can address the cause of plasma disorders by eliminating all endogenous and exogenous toxins, metabolic and decomposition products, and immunological active substances. Consistent implementation of plasmapheresis combined with dialysis and other conventional techniques, may help to improves the as yet poor prognosis for AKI.

Kidney Transplant Rejection

In chronic renal failure, a kidney transplantation is the decisive alternative to permanent dialysis. Rejection of the transplanted kidney is a grave problem. Although various therapeutic interventions to delay or prevent rejection exist and use steroids, immunoglobulins, immunosuppressives, cyclosporine A, tripple drug, OKT3, and other new developed immunosuppressive therapies. Infections and rejection reactions are, the most frequent complications of modern transplantation [101, 102]. Thus, acute kidney transplant rejection is considered as an indication for TA [103, 104]. TA is indicated in the management of rejection crisis due to preformed specific antibodies or a high degree of immunization [105].

Immunological problems like performed donor-specific antibodies or a high degree of immunization complicate the outcome of donor transplantation. Postoperatively the antibody-mediated rejection or drug-related side-effects of the medication can limit the therapeutic success of transplantation. Acute allograft rejection is one of the important complications after renal transplantation, and it is a deleterious factor for long-term graft survival.

Rejection is a complex pathophysiologic process, which has been explained by transcriptome and proteome in RNA transcripts and proteins level respectively [106]. Therefore therapeutic strategies include a primary avoidance of immunization, careful patient selection, a meticulous immunological workup and a proper follow up and therapeutic apheresis as improved therapy [107, 108].

After the blood group barrier had been successfully crossed in Japan in the 1980s, different protocols were developed for ABO-incompatible kidney transplantation and the procedure has gained widespread acceptance and has been implemented in most transplant centers [105, 109-111]. Immunosuppression consists of tacrolimus, mycophenolate and steroids together with induction therapy with an IL-2-receptor blocking agent. The isoagglutinine antibodies against the donor can be eliminated. Firstly, the CD 19/20-positive pre-B cells with a single infusion of rituximab four weeks prior to transplantation and in a second step, the already existing antibodies are depleted by using therapeutic apheresis such as TPE or IA. Novel sensitization and production of antibodies is thereby efficiently prevented [112, 113].

The disadvantage by using TPE is the elimination of physiological proteins, the limitation to 1–1.5 total plasma volume (TPV) as treating dose and the potential for infectious complications such as HIV or hepatitis B or C by using plasma as substitution solution. Therefore various groups use the IA with unselective IgG columns. Patients with performed HLA-antibodies, i.e., a high percentage of panel reactive antibodies, accumulate on the waiting list for kidney transplantation and can experience a substantially longer waiting time [101, 111]. Therefore center specific desensitization protocols were developed in order to transplant these highly immunized patients within a reasonable time frame.

The transplantation procedure is problematic with deceased donor organs as the time for pre-conditioning of the recipient is extremely limited and the accompanying procedures are difficult to perform in time. If transplantation from a living donor with DSA is planned, different protocols were published to desensitize the recipient. These strategies require an intensive procedure, mostly consisting of the administration of intravenous immunoglobulins (IVIG), of intensified immunosuppression, pre- and postoperative TPE or IA and carry a higher risk for antibody-mediated rejection [105, 114-116].

TA in all forms can be applied to remove DSA and multiple HLA antibodies. No selective secondary adsorbers exist, and available columns with a selectivity for immunoglobulins would be considered the best option. Some treatments are usually needed to deplete to recipient of the DSA- and/or anti-HLA titer.

Acute antibody rejection of organ allografts usually presents as severe dysfunction with a high risk of allografts loss. HLA antibodies are involved in AMR [117]. The renal biopsy often cannot rule out one cause or the other with sufficient certainty, leaving the physician with the decision how to treat vascular rejection that can be caused by antibodies or cellular infiltration [118]. TA accompanied by T cell depletion (ATG, ALG, or OKT3) conversion to a tacrolimus-based imunosuppression and pulsed steroids, are used to limit the interstitial and vascular damage [115]. The use of IA targeted against IgG has been used successfully. It is not possible, due to conflicting and limited data, to give general recommendations in regard to the treatment of TPE or IA, the number of apheresis sessions and the best immunosuppressive therapy [119]. A screening for donor-specific antibodies should be performed to monitor the antibody titer during treatment, until 10 sessions with daily treatments initially followed by apheresis every other day can be necessary in a patient with vascular rejection (Banff IIb-III or AMR) [105, 115].

Recurrence or de novo thrombotic microangiopathy (TMA) in the transient patient is observed rarely with the use of calcineurin inhibitors or mTOR inhibitors or acute vascular rejection. Infectious disesases such as HIV, CMV, paravirus B 19, an inhibited or decreased activity of the von Willebrand factor-cleaving metalloprotease ADAMTS13 or mutations in complement receptors may also trigger microangiopathy with either limited or systemic manifestations [105].

TA can be attempted to ameliorate the course of the disease and subsequent graft damage, if switching to a different immunosuppressive regimen or the treatment of an underlying infection does not lead to an improvement of the TMA. The treatment regimen is comparable to TMA in non-transplanted patients. The treated volume is usually one TPV with human albumin and/or fresh frozen plasma as substitution fluid and anticoagulation with heparin on a daily basis until platelet count and lactate dehydrogenase have normalized. Up to 50 percent of patients demonstrate a prompt exacerbation if daily TA is stopped. Continuation of TA on an alternate day strategy for at least two additional treatments can reduce the recurrence rate. Nevertheless TMA reduces graft survival both in recurring or de novo TMA and treatment might not alter the progression of the disease [105].

Goodpasture syndrome or anti-GBM disease can occur de novo in patients following transplantation or as a manifestation of underlying Alport disease, but is rare (e.g., 3 percent of transplanted male Alport patients) [120-122]. The recipient's immune system is exposed to a collagen component carried by the transplanted organ that is lacking in Alport patients and, consequently, the patient might develop antibodies against this antigen in the glomerular basement membrane. These antibodies may then induce post-transplantation anti-GBM disease. The treatment of this condition and of de novo disease is identical to the strategy applied to non-transplanted patients. TA is used in order to remove the causative antibody. Both TPE and IA have been shown to deplete the patient effectively of antibodies and halt disease progression [122, 123]. The TA should be a rapid removal of the antibodies with daily treatments. Treatment frequency should be tapered later to antibody titer measurements. TA is accompanied by an intensified immunosuppressive regimen to suppress further antibody formation [105, 124].

Only few information are available about long-term results of kidney transplantation in adults with focal segmental glomerulosclerosis. But primary FSGS recurs with uncertain incidence after kidney transplantation (presumably 20 percent). A circulating factor is assumed to play a causative role and TA has been successfully applied in patients with recurrent FSGS. In patients treated with a protein-A adsorption column or TPE, a dramatic but usually transient reduction in proteinuria has been observed [123]. This effect was larger with the use of IA, but more prolonged remissions were reported with the use of TPE with or without combination with cyclophosphamide [105, 124].

Therapeutic apheresis in transplantation as an important part of different therapy strategies like for therapy of several conditions such as AMR or ABOi transplantation is accepted today. TA enables the physicians to develop strategies to provide the best organ replacement to patients with high degree of immunization or performed DSA thereby expanding the use of living donation. The standard method has been TPE but it is currently more and more replaced by the more selective methods provided by immunoadsorption. Due to the considerable costs of IA the selection and application of an adsorber and device for IA should be preceded by a judicious effort to characterize and plan the treatment. The specific characteristics of the clinical problem, the capabilities of the choice available and the current evidence have to be known to avoid high costs or inadequate therapy.

The guidelines on the use of TA from the AAC of the ASFA give for the AMR renal transplant recipients and desensitization living donor due to donor specific HLA antibody the category I with the RG 1B. The desensitization high PRA deceased donor has the category III with the RG 2C [6, 7] (Table 1).

The guidelines from the AAC include the barriers to transplantation antibodies to human leukocyte antigens and ABO incompatibility with the donor because there is an increased risk for graft loss secondary to hyperacute rejection of the organ due to endotheial damage. A and B antigens are expressed on vascular endothelium [7]. Patients with elevated HLA antibody screen have difficulty finding an HLA compatible donor and remain on the transplantation list significantly longer than unsensitized patients. The goal of desensitization protocols is to allow these individuals to be transplanted using a donor kidney that would otherwise not be usable due to the high likelihood of graft loss. Allograft rejection has traditionally focused on T cell mediated process causing cellular rejection. Acute vascular rejection has been thought of as antibody mediated based on correlating histological findings with the identification of donor specific antibody. Recently a clear histological diagnosis of antibody-mediated rejection can be made on the Sixth Banff Conference on Allograft pathology in 2001 [6].

AMR affects less than 10 percent of renal allografts. Recipients at increased risk include those with previous transplant and high panel-reactive antibodies [6]. New immunosuppressive drugs are continually being developed to prevent and treat acute allograft rejection. All transplant recipients are placed on immunosuppressive therapy but individuals with a high liklihood of acute rejection, including those with HLA antibodies and recipients of cadaveric organs, receive more intensive regimens. The optimal regimen has yet not to be defined but include the use of cyclosporine, tacrolimus, myocophenolate mofetil, azathioprine, and antilymphocyte globulin [6]. Other monoclonal antibodies are rituximab, bortezomib and eculizumab [7]. The rationale for therapeutic apheresis is that AMR and DSA, which are generated after transplantation, can be removed with TPE, double filtration plasmapheresis, lymphoplasmapheresis, and IA [6]. TPE is used to lower antibody titer below a critical threshold. TPE has been included in preparatory regimes for ABOi renal transplantation in addition to other immuno-suppressive/immunomodulatory drugs Therapies [7]. This is likely due to improved anti-rejections, improved detection of DSA, and improved definition of AMR using the Banff criteria. Previously there was a high graft loss rate with acute vascular rejection, current regimens which include TPE have a graft survival rate of 70–80 percent [6].

TA can also be used prior to transplant to remove HLA antibodies. TPE is used in combination with immunosuppressive drugs pre-transplant until cross-match is negative. TPE is usually continued post-operatively and re-initiated in cases where AMR occurs. The ability to obtain a negative cross-match

depends on the DSA titer. Using approximately 5 TPE pre-operatively, will allow the titer of ≤ 32 to become negative. The risk of AMR is approximately 30 percent with a small number of graft losses. The desensitization protocols should be used only in highly selected patients [6].

Patients should be started on immunosuppressive drugs prior to initiate plasma exchange to limit antibody re-synthesis. For desensitization protocols, there appears to be a correlation between the number of TPE needed pre-operatively to obtain a negative cross-match and the antibody titer [6]. The exchange volume will be 1–1.5 TPV and the replacement fluid can be a human-albumin (5 percent) electrolyte solution. TPE is also performed post-operatively for a minimum of three procedures. Further treatment is determined by risk of AMR, DSA titers, or the occurrence of AMR [6].

Further investigations and more controlled studies will show the importance of TA in the therapy strategies, but the financial aspects of TA are matter of regional negotiation and preference. To simplify reimbursement, transplant centers should define their needs aim for a standard reimbursement and to try to limit price variations of this very expensive therapy [105].

Summary

TA is mostly used by nephrologists due to their extensive training in the management of blood purification methods. Different renal diseases can be treated by various apheresis methods. But there are only a few prospective controlled trials available to allow definitive conclusions. The rationale for TA in HUS is discussed controversially. The treatment strategy is dependent on disease severity. TA and biologic agents, such as eculizumab, in combination seems to be prudent. RPGN is a clinico-pathologic entity consisting of rapid loss of renal function, usually a 50% decline in GFR within some months. Therefore TA is indicated in RPGN (ANCA associated) with dialysis dependence (Cr >6 mg/dL), and in RPGN with diffuse alveolar hemorrhage (anti-glomerular basement membrane disease). TA in RPGN with dialysis independence is only indicated in severe cases if the immunosuppressive therapy has failed. In approximately 60% of patients with RPGN present with crescentic glomerulonephritis (pauci-immune RPGN) with few or absent deposits, some trials have evaluated the efficacy of TA as an adjunct to conventional immunosuppressive therapy. FSGN is caused by a variety of factors, however, one type that recurs after transplantation and has been with

circulating factors, can be treated with TA. MPGN from cryoglobulinemia could be an indication for TA, too. Only in severe cases of myoglobulinemic renal failure TA can be indicated as a supportive therapy. In the inevitable unfavourable prognosis of the AKI therapeutic apheresis can be added to the conservative and extracorporeal therapies, if this therapy failed. TA is indicated in renal transplantation in ABO compatible antibody mediated rejection, desensitization, living donor, and positive crossmatch due to donor specific HLA antibody. In renal transplantation, ABO incompatible, TA is indicated for desensitization live donors and in humoral rejection. But further studies are necessary to prove the benefit of TA in renal diseases.

References

[1]   Bambauer R, Latza R, Schiel R (eds.). Therapeutic Plasma Exchange and Selective Plasma Separation Methods. Fundamental Technologies, Pathology and Clinical Results. 4rd Edition. *Pabst Science Publishers,* Lengerich, 2013.

[2]   De Palo T, Giordano M, Bellantuono R et al. Therapeutic apheresis in children: experience in a pediatric dialysis center. *Int. J. Artif. Org.* 2000, 23(12). 834 – 839.

[3]   Kaplan AA. Why nephrologists should perform therapeutic plasma exchange. *Dial Transplant.* 2009; 38(2): 65 – 70.

[4]   Madore F, Lazarus JM, Brady HR. Therapeutic plasma exchange in renal disease. *J. AM. Soc. Nephrol.* 1996; 7: 367 – 386.

[5]   Bambauer R, C Bambauer, R Latza, R Schiel. Therapeutic apheresis in nephrology. *Clin. Nephrol. Urol. Sci.* 2014, http://www.hoajonline.com/ journals/pdf/2054-7161-1-2.pdf.

[6]   Szczepiorkowski M, Winters J, Bandarenko N et al. Guidelines on the use of therapeutic apheresis in clinical practice-evidence-based approach from the Apheresis Applications Committee of the American Society Apheresis. *J. Clin. Apher.* 2010; 25: 83 -177 (2010).

[7]   Schwartz J, Winters JL, Padmanabhan A et al. Guidlines on the Use of Therapeutic Apheresis in Clinical Practice – Evidence-Based Approach from the Writing Committee of the American Society for Apheresis: The Sixth Special Issue. *J. Clin. Apher.* 2013; 28: 145-284.

[8]   Bambauer R, Schiel R, Lehmann B, Bambauer C. Therapeutic Aphaeresis. Technical Aspects. *ARPN J. Sci. Technol.* 2012; 2: 399-421. http://www.ejournalofscience.org.

[9]   Geigy JR. Scientific tables. In: Diem K, Lentner C, editors. Documenta Geigy: Scientific Tables. 7th ed. Ardsley, NY: *Geigy Pharmazeuticals.* 1970.

[10] Hunt EAK, Jain NG, Somers MJG. Apheresis therapy in children: An overview of key technical aspects and a review of experience in pediatric renal diseases. *J. Clin. Apher.* 2013; 28: 36 – 47.

[11] Michon B, Moghrabi A, Winikoff R et al. Complications of apheresis in children. *Transfusion.* 2007; 47: 1837-1842. doi: 10.1111/j.1537-2995.2007.01405.x.

[12] Bambauer R, Jutzler GA, Philippi H et al. Hemofiltration and plasmapheresis in premature infants and newborns. *Artif. Org.* 1988; 12: 20.

[13] Bambauer R, Latza R, Schiel R. Therapeutic apheresis in the treatment of hemolytic uremic syndrome due to pathophysiologic aspect. *Ther. Apher. Dial.* 2011; 15: 10 – 19.

[14] Zimmerhackl, LB, Verweyen H, Gerber A et al. Das hämolytisch-urämische Syndrom. *Dtsch. Ärztebl.* 2002; 99: A197 – A203.

[15] Spencer CD, Crane FM, Kumar JR et al. Treatment of postpartum haemolytic uremic syndrome with plasma exchange. *JAMA.* 1982; 247: 2808 – 2809.

[16] Gillor A, Roth B, Bulla M et al. Plasmapherese bei der Behandlung von Kindern mit hämolytisch-urämischen Syndrom. *Nieren-Hochdruckkrankh.* 1986; 15: 118 – 123.

[17] Bambauer R, Jutzler GA, Jesberger HJ et al. Therapeutischer Plasma-Austausch beim hämolytisch-urämischen Syndrom. *Dtsch. Med. Wschr.* 1988; 113: 1245 – 1249.

[18] Dittrich E, Schmaldienst S, Derfler K. Plasmaaustausch und Immunadsorption. *Wien. Klin. Wschr. Educ.* 2007; 2: 39 – 54.

[19] Remuzzi G, Marchesi D, Mecca G et al. Haemolytic.uraemic syndrome: Deficiency of plasma factor(s) regulating prostacyclin activity? *Lancet.* 1978; I: 871 – 872.

[20] Kaplan AA. Therapeutic apheresis for cancer related uremic syndrome. *Ther. Apher.* 2001; 4: 201 – 206.

[21] Michael M, Elliot EJ, Ridley GF et al. Interventions for haemolytic uraemia syndrome and thrombotic thrombocytopenic purpura. *Crochane Database Syst. Rev.* 21. Jan. 2009.

[22] O'Regan S, Blais N, Russo P et al. Hemolytic uremic syndrome: glomerular filtration rate, 6 to 11 years later measured by 99mTc DTPA plasma slope clearance. *Clin. Nephrol.* 1989; 32: 217 – 220.

[23] Rasco DA, Webster DR, Sahl JW et al. Origins of the *E. coli* strain causing outbtreak of haemolytic-uremic syndrome in Germany. *N. Eng. J. Med.* 2011; 365: 709 – 717.

[24] Kielstein JT, Beutel G, Feig S et al. Best supportive care and therapeutic plasma exchange with or without eculizumab in Shiga-toxin-producing *E. coli* O104:H4 induced haemolytic-uremic syndrome: an analysis of the German STEC-Hus registry. *Nephrol. Dial Transplant.* 2012; 27(10): 1807 – 1815.

[25] Bach D, Specker C, Horstkotte D et al. Einsatz von Pseudomonas-Immunglobulin auf einer internistischen Intensivstation–zwei Fallberichte. *Intensivmedizin.* 1989; 26:144–148.

[26] Tischer CC and Brenner BM (eds.). Renal pathology with clinical and functional correlation. *J. B. Lippincott,* Philadelphia, USA, 1989.

[27] Klein J and Horejsi V (eds.). Immunology. *Blackwell Science*, Oxford, Berlin, Tokyo, 1997: 348 – 392.

[28] Tao K, Nicholls K, Rockman S and Kincaid-Smith P. Expression of complement 3 receptos (CR1 and CR3) on neutrophils and erythrocytes in patients with IgA nephropathy. *Clin. Nephrol.* 1989; 32: 203-208.

[29] Couser WG. Rapidly progressive glomerulonephritis classification, diseases. *Am. J. Kid Dis.* 1988; 6: 449 -469.

[30] Lin J, Markowitz GS, Valeri AM et al. Renal monoclonal immunoglobulin deposition disease: The disease spectrum. *Am. Soc. Nephrol.* 2001; 12: 1482 – 1492.

[31] Kluth J, Rees AJ. Anti-glomerular basement membrane disease. *J. Am. Soc. Nephrol.* 1999; 10: 2446 – 2453.

[32] Wieslander J, Byrgen P, Heinegard D. Isolation of the specific glomerular basement membrane antigen involved in Goodpasture syndrome. *Proc. Natl. Acad. Sci..* 1984; 81: 1544 – 1549.

[33] Müller GA, Seipl L, Risler T. Treatment of non anti-GNM-antibody mediated rapidly progressive glomerulonephritis by plasmapheresis and immunosuppression. *Klin. Wschr.* 1989; 64: 140 – 147.

[34] Risler T. Therapie der Glomerulonephritis? *Mitt. Klin. Nephrol.* 1992; 21: 26 – 33.

[35] Lockwood CM. Controlled trial of plasma-exchange in non-antibody-mediated rapidly progressive glomerulonephritis. *Annales de Medicine.* 1984; 135 – 137.

[36] Siebert HG. Stellenwert der Plasmaseparation zur Behandlung von Nierenerkrankungen. *Mitt. Klin. Nephrol.* 1983; 12: 19 – 36.

[37] Jayne DRW, Gaskin G, Rasmussen N et al. European Vasculitis Study Group. Randomized trial of plasma exchange or high-dosage methylprednisolone as adjunctive therapy for severe renal vasculitis. *J. Am. Soc. Nephrol.* 2007; 18: 2188 – 2188.

[38] Harada T, Ozono Y, Miyazaki M et al. Plasmapheresis in the treatment of rapidly progressive glomerulonephritis. *Ther. Apher.* 1997; 1: 366 – 369.

[39] Kaplan AA. Core cirriculum in Nephrology. Therapeutic Plasma Exchange. Core Curriculum 2008. *Am. J. Kid Dis.* 2008; 52: 1180 – 1196.

[40] De Lind van Wingaarden RA, Hauer HA, Wolterbeck R et al. Clinical and histologic determinants of renal outcome in ANCA-associated vasculitis: A prospective analysis of 10 patients with severe renal involvement. *J. Am. Soc. Nephrol.* 2006; 17: 2264 – 2272.

[41] De Lind van Wingaarden RA, Hauer HA, Wolterbeck R et al. for the European Vasculitis Study Group (EUVAS). Changes of renal recovery for dialysis-dependent ANCA-associated glomerulonephritis. *J. Am. Soc. Nephrol.* 2007; 18: 2189 – 2189.

[42] Johnson JP, Moore JJ, Austin HA et al. Therapy of anti-glomerular basement membrane antibody disease: Analysis of prognostic significance of clinical, pathologic and treatment factors. *Medicine.* 1985; 64: 219 – 227.

[43] Brusselle GG. Pulmonary-renal syndromes. *Acta Clin. Belg.* 2007; 63: 88 – 96.

[44] Levy JB, Hammad T, Coulthard A et al. Clinical features and outcomes of patients with both ANCA and anti-GBM antibodies. *Kid. Int.* 2004; 66: 1535 – 1540.

[45] Sanchez PS, Ward DM. Therpaeutic apheresis for renal disorders. *Sem. Dial.* 2012; 25: 119 – 131.

[46] Sinha SA, Tiwari AN, Chanchlani R et al. Therapeutic plasmapheresis using membrane plasma separation. *India J. Pediat.* 2012; 79(8): 1084 – 1086.

[47] Stegmayr B, Abdel-Rahman EM, Balogun RA. Septic shock with multiorgan failure: from conventional apheresis to adsorption therapies. *Sem. Dial.* 2012: 24: 171 – 175.

[48] Walsh M, Casian A, Flossmann O et al. Long-term follow-up of patients with severe ANCA-associated vasculitis comparing plasma exchange to intravenous methylprednisolone treatment is unclear. *Kid. Int.*.2013; 84: 397 - 402.

[49] Guo S, Mühlfeld AS, Wietecha TA et al. Deletion of acting Fcγ receptors does not confer protection in murine cryoglobulinemia-associated membranoproliferative glomerulonephritis. *Am. J. Pathol.* 2009; 175: 107 – 116.

[50] Clynes R, Dumitru C, Ravetch JV. Uncouplin of immune complex formation and kidney damage in autoimmune glomerulonaphritis. *Science.* 1998; 279: 1052 – 1054.

[51] Sieberth HG, Maurin N. The therapy of rapidly progressive glomerulonephritis. *Klin. Wschr.* 1983; 61: 1001 – 1010.

[52] Matic G, Hofmann D, Winkler R et al. Removal of immunoglobulins by protein A versus an anti-human immunoglobulin G-based system: Evaluation of 602 sessions of extracorporeal immunoadsorption. *Artif. Org.* 2000; 24: 103 – 107.

[53] Pusey CD, Levy JB. Plasmapheresis in immunologic renal disease. *Blood Purif.* 2012; 33(1-3): 190 – 198.

[54] Hasegawa M, Kawamura N, Kasugai M et al. Cytapheresis for the treatment of myeloperoxidase antineutrophil cytoplasmatic anti-associated vasculitis: Report of 5 cases. *Ther. Apher.* 2002; 6: 443 – 449.

[55] Cole E, Caffran D, Magli A. A prospective randomised trial of plasma exchange as additive therapy in idiopathic crescentic glomerulonephritis. The Canadian Aphersis Study Group. *Am. J. Kid Dis.* 1992; 20: 261 – 270.

[56] Riffle G, Dechette E. Treatment of rapidly progressive glomerulonephritis by plasma exchange and methylprednisolone pulses. A prospective randomized trial cyclophosphamide interim analysis. The French Cooperative Group. *Prog. Clin. Biol. Res.* 1990; 337: 263 – 270.

[57] Palmer A, Cairns T, Dische F et al. Treatment of rapidly progressive glomerulonephritis extracorporeal immunoadsorption, prednisolone and cyclophosphamide. *Nephrol. Dial. Transplant.* 1991; 6: 536 – 542.

[58] Stegmayr BG Almroth G, Berlin G et al. Plasma exchange or immunoadsorption in patients with rapidly ptogressive crescentic glomerulonephritis. A Swedish multi-center study. *Int. J. Artif. Org.* 1999; 22: 81 – 87.

[59] Cascian AL, Jayne DRW. Role of plasma exchange in the treatment of primary vasculitis. *Int. J. Clin. Rheumatol.* 2010; 5: 339 – 344.

[60] Hayes JS, Chang J, Abdel-Rahman EM. Therapeutic plasma exchange for related conditions in the elderly: Ten years experience in one center. *Sem. Dial.* 2012; 25: 159 – 164.

[61] Walsh M, Catapano F, Szpirt W et al. Plasma exchange for renal vasculitis and idiopathic rapidly progressive glomerulonephritis: A meta-analysis. *Am. J. Kid. Dis.* 2011; 57(4): 566 – 574.

[62] Paczek L, Teschner mM, Schaeffer RM et al. Intraglomerular proteolytic enzymes in Heymann nephritis. *J. Nephrol.* 1991; 4: 221 – 228.

[63] Strutz F, Lueg HO, Risler T et al. Proteinurie und atherogenes Risiko. *Dtsch. Med. Wschr.* 1992; 117: 1267 – 1272.

[64] Gans ROB, Brentjens JRH, Donker AJM. Therapeutic approach to nephritis syndrome. *J. Nephrol.* 1990; 2: 117 – 122.

[65] Palla, R Cirami, C, Panichi V et al. Intravenous immunoglobulin therapy of membranous nephropathy: efficacy and safety. *Clin. Nephrol.* 1991; 35: 98 – 104.

[66] Bagga A, Hari P, Moudgil A. Mycophenolate mofetil and prednisolone therapy in children with steroid-dependent nephritic syndrome. *Am. J. Kid Dis.* 2003; 42: 1114 – 1120.

[67] Bagga A Mantan M. Nephrotic syndrome in children. *Ind. J. Med. Red.* 2005; 120: 13 – 19.

[68] Habashy D, Hodson EM, Craig JC. Interventions for steroid-resistant nephritic syndrome: a systemic review. *Pediatr. Nephrol.* 2004; 18: 906 – 912.

[69] Burgharg R, Klein W, Leititis JU et al. Cycosporin A (CyA) treated of nephrotic syndrome (NS) in children. *Am. Soc. Nephrol.* 1987; 38: A25 – A32.

[70] Kashtan C, Melvin T, Kim Y. Long-term follow-up of patients with steroid-dependent minimal change glomerulonephrits. *Clin. Nephrol.* 1988; 29: 79 – 85.

[71] Briggs WA, Choi MJ, Scheel PJ. Successful mycophenolate mofetil treatment of glomerular disease. *Am. J. Kid Dis.* 1998; 32: 213 – 217.

[72] Cattran DC, Wang MM, Appel G et al. Mycophenolate mofetil in the treatment of focal segmental glomerulonephritis. *Clin. Nephrol.* 2004; 62: 405 – 411.

[73] Mc Cauly J, Tzakis AG, Fung JJ et al. FK 506 in steroid-resistant focal sclerosing glomerulonephritis in childhood. *Lancet.* 1990; 335: 674 – 675.

[74] Hirasawa H, Sugai T, Oda T et al. Efficacy and limition of apheresis therapy in critical care. *Ther. Apher.* 1997; 1: 228 – 232.

[75] Savin VJ, Sharma R, Sharma M et al. Circulating factor associated with increased glomerular permeability to albumin in recurrent focal segmental. *N. Engl. J. Med.* 1996; 334: 878 – 883.

[76] Haas, M, Godfin Y, Oberbauer R et al. Plasma immunoadsorption treatment in patients with primary focal and segmental gloemerulonephritis. *Nephrol. Dial Transplant.* 1998; 13: 2013 – 2017.

[77] Ronco, PM, Alyanakian, MA Mougenot B. legit chain deposition disease: A model of glomerulosclerosis defined at the molecular level. *Am. Soc. Nephrol.* 2001; 12: 1558 – 1565.

[78] Dantal J, Bigot E, Boges W et al. Effect of plasma protein adsorption on protein excretion in kidney-transplant recipients with recurrent nephritic syndrome. *N. Engl. J. Med.* 1994; 330: 7 – 14.

[79] Tune BM, Mendoza SA. Treatment of idiopathic nephritic syndrome: Regimens and outcomes in children and adults. *J. Am. Soc. Nephrol.* 1997; 8: 824 – 829.

[80] Müller GA, Rodemann HP. Untersuchungen zur in vitro Proliferation von Fibroblasten, etabliert aus mit interstitieller Fibrose. *Mitt. Klin. Nephrol.* 1991; 20: 29 – 36.

[81] Matto TK, Mahmoud MA. Increased maintenance corticosteroids during upper respiratory infection decrease the risk of relapse in nephritic syndrome. *Nephron.* 2000; 85: 342 – 348.

[82] Nakayama M, Katafuchi R, Yanase T et al. Steroid responsiveness and frequency of relapse in adult – onset minimal change nephrotic syndrome. *Am. J. Kid Dis.* 2002; 39: 503 – 512.

[83] Musco E, Mune M, Fujii Y et al. The Kansai FGS LDL-Apheresis Treatment (K-FLAT) Study Group. *Nephron.* 2001; 89: 408 – 414.

[84] Alshaya HO, Al Maghrabi JA, Kari JA. Intravenous pulse cyclophosphamide – is it effective in children with steroid-resistant nephrotic syndrome? *Pediatr. Nephrol.* 2006; 18: 1143 – 1146.

[85] Schifferli J, Favre H, Nydegger U et al. High-dose intravenous IgG treatment and renal function. *Lancet.* 1991; 337: 457 – 458.

[86] Dantal J, Godfrin Y, Koll R et al. Antihuman immunoglobulin affinity immunoadsorption strongly decreases proteinuria in patients with relapsing nephritic syndrome. *J. Am. Soc. Nephrol.* 1998; 9: 1709 – 1715.

[87] Esnault VL, Besnier D, Testa A, et al. Effect of protein A immunoadsorption in nephrotic syndrome of various etiologies. *J. Am. Soc. Nephrol.* 1999; 20: 2014 – 2017.

[88] Russo GE, Bonello M, Bauco B et al. Nephrotic syndrome and plasmapheresis. *Int. J. Art. Org.* 1999; 23: 111 – 117.

[89] Hattori M, Chikamoto H, Akioka Y et al. A combined low-density lipoprotein apheresis and prednisone therapy for steroid-resistant primary focal segmental glomerulosclerosis in children. *Am. J. Kid Dis.* 2003; 42: 1121 – 1130.

[90] Russel TA. Acute renal failure related to rhabdomyolysis: pathophysiology, diagnosis, and collaborative management. *Nephrol. Nurs. J.* 2000; 27: 567 – 575.

[91] Criddle LA. Rabdomyolysis. *Crit. Care Nurse.* 2003; 23: 14 – 30.

[92] Fumagalli MM, Bruzzone DV, Diana CA et al. Rhabdomyolitic acute renal failure in cardiac surgery: A clinical case. *Miner. Anesthesiol.* 1995; 61: 937 – 941.

[93] Siebenlist D, Kobe R, Gartenlöhner W. Plasmapherese in der Therapie des myoglobulinämischen Nierenversagens. *Intensivmedizin.* 1993; 30: 15 – 19.

[94] Yang KC, Su TC, Lee YT. Treatment of fibrate-induced rhabdomyolysis with plasma exchange in ESRD. *Am. J. Kid Dis.* 2005; 45: e57 – 59.

[95] Ronco C. Extracorporeal therapies in acute rhabdomyolysis and myoglobin clearance. *Crit. Care.* 2005; 9: 141 – 142.

[96] Swaroop R, Zabaneh R, Parimoo N. Plasmapheresis in a patient with rhabdomyolysis: case report. *Cases J.* 2009; 2: 215 – 218.

[97] Rubanyi GM, Guillaume JC, Revuz J et al. The role of endothelium on cardiovascular homeostasis and diseases. *Cardiovasc. Pharmacol.* 1994; 2 (Suppl. 4): S1 – S14.

[98] Bambauer R. New approaches in the treatment of acute kidney injury. *Ther. Apher. Dial.* 2009; 13: 248 – 253.

[99] Kribben A. Pathogenese des akuten Nierenversagens. *Mitt. Klin. Nephrol.* 2004; XXXIII: 33 – 35.

[100] Cameron S, Davison AM, Grünfeld JP et al. (eds.). Oxford Textbook of Clinical Nephrology. *University Press Oxford*, Oxford, New York, Tokyo, 1992.

[101] Fischer JE, Kirstle G, Blümke M. OKT 3-Dosis-Reduktion als effektives Therapeutikum steroidresistenter Abstoßungen nach Nierentransplantation. *Nieren- Hochdruckkrankh.* 1991; 20: 8 – 12.

[102] Kaczmarek I, Deutsch MA, Sadoni S et al. Successful management of antibody-mediated cardiac allograft rejection with combined immunoadsorption and anti-CD20 monoclonal antibody treatment: Case

report and literature report. *J. Heart Lung Transplant.* 2007; 26: 511 –
515.

[103] Cueller-Cabera H, Ramirez-Fernandez M, Guerra-Rosales MJ et al.
Plasmapheresis, immunosuppressive therapy and kidney transplantation
in a pre-sensitized patient. *Bol. Med. Hosp. Mex.* 1989; 46: 246 – 251.

[104] Schwenger V, Morath C. Immunoadsorption in nephrology and kidney
transplantation. *Nephrol. Dial Transplant.* 2010; 25(8): 2407 – 2413.

[105] Teschner S, Kurschat C, Burst V. Therapeutic apheresis in
transplantation: overview and critical evaluation of available modalities
in respect to indications, evidence and costs. *Transplantationsmedizin.*
2010; 22: 266 – 272.

[106] Mao Y, Bai J, Chen J. A pilot study of GC/MS-based serum metallic
profiling of acute rejection in renal transplantation. *Transplant.
Immunol.* 2008; 19: 74 – 79.

[107] Gloor JM, Winters JL, Cornell LD et al. Baseline donor-specific
antibody levels and outcomes in positive cross-match kidney
transplantation. *Am. J. Transplant.* 2010; 10: 582 – 588.

[108] Ichimaru N, Takahara S. Japan´s experience with living-donor kidney
transplantation across ABO barriers. *Nat. Clin. Pract. Nephrol.* 2008; 4:
682 – 692.

[109] Sawada T, Fuchinoue S, Teraoka S. Successful A1-to O ABO-
incompatibility kidney transplantation after a preconditioning regimen
consisting of anti-CD20 monoclonal antibody infusions, splenectomy,
and double filtration. *Transplantation.* 2009; 74: 1207 – 1214.

[110] Donauer J, Wilpert J, Geyer M et al. ABO-incompatible kidney
transplantation using antigen-specific immunoadsorption and rituximab:
a single center experience. *Xenotransplantation.* 2006; 13: 108 – 114.

[111] Scharma A, Bummerts J, Gomez-Navarro D et al. Clearance for
monoclonal antibody (mab) CP-675,206 by therapeutic plasma exchange
(TPE) or plasmapheresis. *J. Clin. Oncol.* 2007; 25 (Suppl.): 1515 –
1519.

[112] Franz HJC, Rahmel A, Doxiadis IIL. Enhanced kidney allocation to
highly sensitized patients by a acceptable mismatch program.
*Transplantation.*2009; 88: 447 – 452.

[113] Gloor JM, DeGoey SR, Pineda AA. Overcoming a positive cross-match
in liver donor kidney transplantation. *Am. J. Transplant.* 2003; 3: 1017 –
1022.

[114] Jordan SC, Tyan D, Stablein D et al. Evaluation of intravenous immunoglobulin as an agent to lower allosensitization and improve transplantation in highly sensitized adult patients with end-stage renal disease: report of the NIH IG02 trial. *J. Am. Soc. Nephrol.* 2004; 15: 3256 – 3262.

[115] Vo A, Lukowsky M, Toyoda M et al. Rituximab and intravenous immune globulin for desensitization during renal transplantation. *N. Engl. J. Med.* 2008; 359: 242 – 248.

[116] Venetz JP, Pascual M. New treatments for acute humoral rejection of kidney allografts. *Inform. Healthca.* 2007; 16: 625 – 631.

[117] Higgins R, Zehnder D, Chen J. The histological development of acute antibody-mediated rejection in HLA antibody-incompatible renal transplantation. *Nephrol. Dial. Transplant.* 2010; 25: 1306 – 1312.

[118] Takemoto SK, Zevi A, Feng S. National conference to assess antibody-mediated rejection in solid organ transplantation. *Am. J. Transplant.* 2004; 4: 1033 – 141.

[119] Böhmig GA, Wahrmann M, Regele H et al. Immunoadsorption in severe C4d-positive acute kidney allograft rejection: a randomized controlled trial. *Q. Am. J. Transplant.* 2001; 7: 117 – 122.

[120] Byrne MC, Budisavljevic MN, Fan Z et al. Renal transplant in patients with Alport´s syndrome. *Am. J. Kid. Dis.* 2002; 39: 769 – 775.

[121] Laczika K, Knapp S, Derfler K et al. Immunoadsorption in Goodpasture´s syndrome. *Am. J. Kid. Dis.* 2000; 36: 392 – 395.

[122] Bolton WK. Goodpasture´s syndrome. *Kid Int*.1996; 50: 1753 – 1759.

[123] Dantal J, Bigot E, Bogers W et al. Effect of plasma protein adsorption on protein excretion in kidney-transplant recipients with recurrent nephritic syndrome. *N. Engl. J. Med.* 1994; 330: 7 – 14.

[124] DallAmico R, Ghiggeri G, Carraro M et al. Prediction and treatment of recurrent focal segmental glomerulosclerosis after renal transplantation in children. *Am. J. Kid Dis.* 1999; 34: 1048 – 1055.

In: Hemolytic Uremic Syndrome   ISBN: 978-1-63463-227-0
Editors: Glenna Clayton   © 2015 Nova Science Publishers, Inc.

Chapter III

The Consequences of Soliris® Therapy in Patients with aHUS

Karin Janssen van Doorn, M.D. [*]

Nephrology Department, University Hospital Antwerp, Belgium

Abstract

Atypical HUS (aHUS) is a sub-type of Hemolytic Uremic Syndrome in which the origin of the thrombotic micro-angiopathy (TMA) is the result of a decreased regulation of the alternative complement pathway on cell surfaces due to a genetic cause. aHUS is a rare disease that, despite the standard treatment with plasmapheresis, often progresses to terminal renal failure with associated co-morbidity, such as long term renal replacement therapy (RRT). As such, aHUS has a poor prognosis and is associated with high morbidity and mortality.

The complement system plays a key role in the induction of endothelial damage in patients with aHUS. Recent advances in genetic research demonstrate that mutations in the genes that code for complement factors provoke the induction of endothelial damage. The observation that excessive activation of the alternative pathway of complement underlies the pathogenesis of aHUS seems to make clear that the complement inhibition is the crux of the treatment.

[*] Corresponding author: Karin Janssen van Doorn, MD. Nephrology Department, University Hospital Antwerp, Belgium. E-mail: k.janssenvandoorn@gmail.com.

Eculizumab (Soliris®) is a monoclonal antibody (anti-C5) that inhibits the terminal fraction of the complement system, by blocking the formation of a cell membrane attack complex and C5a. It is well known that eculizumab involves an interruption of the TMA process.

Eculizumab was first introduced as treatment of paroxysmal nocturnal hemoglobinuria and seemed also effective in the treatment of plasmapheresis resistant aHUS. Therefore, in 2011 both the US Food and Drug Administration (FDA) and the European Medicines Agency (EMA) approved the use of eculizumab to treat aHUS.

Eculizumab improves renal function not only in early treated patients without need of RRT, but also in patients with RRT, which implies an improvement of health related quality of life.

In other words, eculizumab should be initiated as early as feasible in order to optimize the recovery of renal function, and should also be used in patients after renal transplantation when it seems certain that an underlying aHUS could relapse.

In contrast, Soliris® should be permanently recommended to patients, unless discontinuation of Soliris® is clinically indicated. However, therapy with Soliris® is expensive and the administration is subject to several conditions. Eculizumab is not without risks, being associated with the development of meningococcal disease. That means all patients should be vaccinated before the onset of treatment and should in addition receive prophylactic antibiotics.

Furthermore, a lifetime intake of immunosuppressive therapy has a considerable impact on a patient's quality of life.

To conclude, the administration of eculizumab has serious advantages for a patient's personal life and social interest in general.

Background

Hemolytic uremic syndrome (HUS) is characterized by the triad non-immune micro-angiopathic hemolytic anemia, thrombocytopenia and acute renal failure, mostly presenting in childhood following an episode of diarrhea, caused by Shiga-like toxin-producing organisms. The atypical, non-diarrheal form (aHUS) can be familial or sporadic, and is associated with several underlying predisposing factors, such as autoimmune systemic diseases, neoplasm, pregnancy, HIV and certain medications [1-3].

Histological damage from HUS is characterized by the appearance of systemic thrombotic micro-angiopathy (TMA), which primarily affects the renal blood vessels, producing thickening of the vessel wall, thrombosis and obstruction of the vascular lumen. The initial onset of this disease can be abrupt, although it may occur progressively in approximately 20% of patients. High levels of lactate dehydrogenase, undetectable haptoglobin levels, and schistocytes confirm the presence of intravascular hemolysis. Patients develop hematuria, proteinuria, and/or acute renal failure, often accompanied with hypertension, due to volume overload or vascular damage [3].

Although, aHUS predominantly affects the renal vessels, the diffuse character of TMA leads to involvement of the microvasculature of other organ systems, which explains the common appearance of extra-renal symptoms [3].

aHUS is considered a rare disease with an annual incidence rate of 1-2 cases/million inhabitants in the United States and in Europe 3.3 patients/ million inhabitants/year in individuals younger than 18 years of age, with lower rates in adults [2, 3]. This extremely low incidence rate and the specific niche of this disease have implications for the development of pharmaceutical treatment options.

The Role of Complement in aHUS

However, advances in the past 15 years have shown that aHUS is a disorder of the alternative pathway of complement.

Complement consists of multiple plasma and membrane-bound proteins, which trigger several pathways of enzymatic reactions designed for opsonization of pathologic targets, promotion of inflammatory and immune responses and promotion of anaphylatoxins release. The complement system is essential in the defense against infection, the processing of immune complexes, the antibody responses and the elimination of cell remnants from apoptosis.

It is activated by three pathways: the classical, lectin and alternative pathway. All three converge at the point of cleavage of C3. C3 is cleaved by the C3 convertase, into C3b and C3a. C3b binds indiscriminately to pathogens and host cells and its deposition on an antigen mark it for adherence and consequent elimination by phagocytic cells. In addition, C3b exponentially amplifies the activation of the complement system, promoting the formation of more C3-convertase.

The alternative pathway is continuously activated at a low level. In order to avoid complete consumption by the activation of the complement system as well as damage to untargeted tissues (C3b binds indiscriminately to both pathogenic cells and native somatic cells), a number of regulatory proteins act to dissociate the C3-convertase and induce the degradation of C3b.

Key factors of this pathway are factor B (CFB), factor H (CFH), factor I (CFI), thrombomodulin and membrane cofactor protein (MCP).

All factors operate at different levels of the pathway and control the spontaneous activity of C3 convertase [2, 4]. In some patients, the presence of an autoantibody, the C3 nephritic factor (C3NeF), interferes with these normal regulatory mechanisms [2]. Mutations in the complement regulatory proteins CFH, CFI, and MCP and complement CFB and C3, all result in complement over activation [5-8].

The activation of the alternative pathway occurs under normal conditions in a tightly regulated, sequential manner and deposition is limited to those structures responsible for the activation [1, 3, 9-11].

Typically for aHUS is a chronic, uncontrolled complement activity. Multiple studies have reported that 40-60% of patients with aHUS carry mutations in the complement system genes [(complement factor H gene (CFH), the CFH gene cluster, membrane cofactor protein gene (MCP), complement factor I (CFI), thrombomodulin (THBD), complement factor B gene (CFB) and C3 gene (C3)], which are related to deregulation of the alternative pathway. Genetic defects and/or mutations in activators and/or inhibitors lead to chronic activity of the complement system, causing endothelial cell damage and continuous platelet aggregation.

Recent research into the genetic component of aHUS (including the identification of multiple mutations and polymorphisms in the genes that code for certain complement proteins) has led to the conclusion that the endothelial damage produced by the complement system is the critical factor in the pathophysiology of the disease [3]. Moreover, due to a genetic deficiency of complement regulators, aHUS is a permanent, ongoing disease of systemic, complement-mediated thrombotic micro-angiopathy (TMA) [1, 9]. Besides, complement-amplifying conditions place patients with aHUS at high risk for TMA manifestations and may unmask aHUS [12].

Not only mutations, but also anti-FH auto-antibodies directed towards the C-terminal region are found in 5-10% of all patients with aHUS, with similar consequences to those produced by FH mutations [3].

Penetrance of aHUS in carriers of mutations in the complement genes is approximately 50%. Usually in families with complement mutations only some carriers develop aHUS with variable clinical presentations. There is also a wide range of clinical heterogeneity between unrelated patients with the same mutation. This suggests that additional genetic and environmental factors exist and modulate the development and progression of this disease. Polymorphism and the fact that as many as 10% of patients with aHUS have mutations in more than one complement gene, indicates that the coincidence of different genetic risk factors is a determining factor in the development of aHUS (multiple hit theory) [3].

Genetic mutation cannot be identified in 30% - 50% of patients with aHUS [9]. Interestingly, the clinical evolution of patients with aHUS is influenced by the type of mutation involved. In general, patients with FH and C3 mutations have a worse prognosis during the episode of aHUS and following months, with rates of mortality and end stage renal disease (ESRD) or recurrence of 50% - 70% and 50% respectively. On the other hand, only 0.6% of patients with MCP mutations die or develop ESRD, although the risk of recurrence is greater. Seventy-five percent of patients with FH, C3 or FB mutations die or develop ESRD [3].

Limitations of Supportive Care Options

Until recently only plasma therapy (plasma infusion (PI) or plasma exchange (PE)) was available as supportive care during a manifestation of aHUS. PI involves vitro inactive, non-native, fresh frozen plasma (FFP) with functional complement regulators. In PE, the patient receives FFP to replace the native plasma with aHUS, which implies the administration of not only elevated levels of functional complement regulatory proteins, but also the elimination of dysfunctional endogenic soluble complement inhibitors together with a lower risk of volume overload. In addition, PE purifies the blood of anti-FH antibodies and the possible presence of inflammatory/thrombogenic factors that participate in producing endothelial damage and platelet hyper-aggregation. Although information from prospective clinical trials is not available, the treatment of choice for episodes of aHUS consisted of early and intensive PE at high volumes and variable frequency based on disease activity. Normally plasma therapy is not considered effective in patients with MCP mutations, since this is a non-circulation protein anchored in the cell membrane, and virtually all of these patients go into remission after the episode of aHUS, regardless of the use of plasma therapy [3, 8].

The rates of complete hematological and renal recovery in patients treated with plasma therapy are lower than 50% (except patients with ESRD and MCP mutations) and these rates are extremely low in patients with FH and FI mutations (5% and 12.5%) [9].

Certain observations indicate that early and intensive PE is essential for protecting patients from aHUS, and PE can prevent disease recurrence and ESRD [13-15].

The results of kidney transplantation in patients with ESRD according to aHUS are limited and depend of the type of mutation. There is a high percentage of post-transplant recurrence of the disease which leads to graft loss [3, 15]. Besides, kidney transplantation is associated with an unacceptable risk of very high morbidity and mortality [2, 16, 17].

Another proposed therapy consists of combined kidney-liver transplantation, which remains, however, a high-risk procedure [18].

Eculizumab

It seems clear that inhibition of the complement system is a viable treatment option in patients with aHUS. In 2011, governing regulatory agencies of the United States and Europe approved the indication for eculizumab (Soliris[®]; Alexion Pharmaceuticals, Connecticut, US), a humanized monoclonal antibody that inhibits the activation of C5 and blocks the generation of the pro-inflammatory anaphylotoxin C5a and the membrane attack complex (C5b-9) of the complement system (which produces cell lysis), for the treatment of aHUS [3].

Eculizumab was first discovered and developed for the rare hemolytic disease paroxysmal nocturnal hemoglobinuria (PNH). In this disease somatic mutations result in a deficiency of glycosylphosphatidylinositol-linked surface proteins, including the terminal complement inhibitor CD59, on hematopoietic stem cells. In a dysfunctional bone marrow background, these mutated progenitor blood cells expand and populate the periphery. Deficiency of CD59 on PHN red blood cells results in chronic complement-mediated intravascular hemolysis, a process central in the morbidity and mortality of PHN.

A recently developed, humanized monoclonal antibody directed against complement component C5; eculizumab blocks the pro-inflammatory and cytolytic effects of terminal complement activation. The approval of eculizumab as a first in class complement inhibitor for the treatment of PNH validates the concept of complement inhibition as an effective therapy and

suppression therapy should be administrated as a concom
patients with aHUS anti-FH antibodies. The response to treatm
s should be monitored through the evolution of antibody titres [3
h not necessary for the clinical diagnosis of aHUS, a complet
of the complement system is recommended, including plasma
complement factors and a complete genetic analysis of affected
wever, a genetic diagnosis of abnormal complement genes would
sessing prognosis on an individual basis, as well as the risk of
f the disease, making this a recommended step for all patients.
ts who are potential candidates for kidney transplantation, the
sis is indispensable [3].
of childbearing potential have to use effective contraception
ent and up to 5 months after treatment. For Soliris®, no clinical
sed pregnancies are available. Human IgG are known to cross the
ntal barrier, and thus eculizumab may potentially cause terminal
inhibition in the fetal circulation and causes fetal morbidity.
oliris® should be given to a pregnant woman only if clearly
unknown whether eculizumab is excreted into human milk. Since
al products and immunoglobulins are secreted into human milk,
of the potential for serious adverse reactions in nursing infants,
g should be discontinued during treatment and up to 5 months
t (Alexion; Soliris® leaflet).

Ethical Annotation

dy written above, aHUS has an annual incidence rate of 1 - 3
inhabitants' individuals younger than 18 years of age, with lower
s. This means, aHUS is considered to be a rare disease, affecting
ifferent age categories but adequate treatment is available for
egory. The drug eculizumab, is a product of niche marketing and
very expensive. Eculizumab is not available to everyone and is
der strict recommendation.
less, eculizumab is a young drug and therefore information of
ake and the achievable adverse events are still not available. The
tious complications by *Neisseria*, and the genetic screening for
heir relatives needs further ethical investigation.

provided rationale for investigation of other indications, such as aHUS in which complement plays a role [19].

The safety profile of eculizumab for patients with aHUS was generally consistent with that in a study involving patients with paroxysmal nocturnal hemoglobinuria who received treatment for up to 8 years [22].

The efficacy and safety of eculizumab as a treatment for aHUS was evaluated in two prospective studies, and the response to eculizumab was similar between patients with mutations and/or anti-FH antibodies and those with no genetic abnormalities. The response was also similar regardless of the type of mutation identified. After six months of treatment with eculizumab, rates of hematological normalization reached 76% in resistant cases and 90% in chronic cases. Eculizumab was associated with significant increases in the estimated glomerular filtration rate (eGFR).

Earlier intervention with eculizumab was associated with significantly greater improvement in the eGFR. Eculizumab was also associated with improvement in health-related quality of life. No cumulative toxicity of therapy or serious infection-related adverse events, including meningococcal infections, were observed through the extension period.

After one year of eculizumab treatment, proteinuria levels were significantly lower than baseline values. Adverse side effects were peritonitis, influenza infection, venous disorder and severe hypertension.

Except for severe hypertension (this patient was already known with hypertension) all adverse events were possibly or probably drug-related. All serious adverse events possibly or probably related to eculizumab resolved without interruption of treatment.

Adverse events were similar among patient subgroups, including the patients who had undergone kidney transplantation and were receiving concomitant immunosuppressive therapy. Eculizumab increases the risk of infection by *Neisseria Meningitidis,* which prompted the vaccination of all patients against *Neisseria* before starting treatment or antibiotic prophylaxis, with no cases of meningitis produced. Survival was 100% [3, 20].

In a French retrospective study of adult patients with aHUS receiving eculizumab, 4 or more weekly 900 mg infusions, the risk of reaching ESRD within 3 months and 1 year of aHUS onset were reduced by half in eculizumab-treated patients compared with recent historical controls [21].

Several cases with other diseases or rare manifestations of aHUS and positive results after eculizumab treatment already have been published [23-26]. Knowledge of the use of eculizumab preventing or treating aHUS in the post-transplant settings, according to individualized recurrence risk assessment is limited. One prospective study followed 22 renal transplant recipients with aHUS who received off-label therapy with anti-C5. Nine patients, all carrying a complement genetic abnormality associated with a high risk of aHUS recurrence, received prophylactic eculizumab to prevent post-transplant recurrence. Eight of them had a successful recurrence-free post-transplant course and achieved a satisfactory graft function, while the remaining patient experienced early arterial thrombosis of the graft.

Thirteen renal transplant recipients were given eculizumab for post-transplant aHUS recurrence. A complete reversal of aHUS activity was obtained in all of them. Importantly, the delay of eculizumab initiation after the onset of the aHUS episode inversely correlated with the degree of renal function improvement. The patients in whom anti-C5 was subsequently stopped experienced a relapse. These data suggest that long-term eculizumab is highly effective for preventing and treating post-transplant aHUS recurrence and indicates that treatment with anti-C5 should be promptly started if a recurrence occurs [27]. Whether it will be safe to withdraw eculizumab in these patients after several years is not yet known.

Treatment

Early and intensive PE should be administrated until eculizumab is an available option. PE and FFP should be preferentially evaluated (1.5 per volume plasma (60 - 75ml/kg) per session. Sessions should be continued until platelet levels have normalized, hemolysis has stopped and a sustained improvement in renal function has been observed for several days. Later (sessions/week should be administered during the following 2 weeks, followed by another two weeks of 3 sessions per week and an individualized assessment for considering the appropriateness of continued treatment [3].

Prior to this point, it is necessary to vaccinate all patients against *Neisseria meningitides*. (Preferably with conjugated tetravalent vaccines against serotypes A, C, Y and W135).

In case that treatment with eculizumab cannot be delayed until obtaining vaccination, treatment can still be started along with antibiotic prophylaxis against *Neisseria meningitides*. In pediatric patients, vaccination against *Haemophilus influenza* and pneumococci is also necessary [3].

When a patient presents with features compatible with a diagnosis of aHUS, the following investigations should be undertaken to exclude other

causes of a TMA: ADAMTS13 activity (TT coli endotoxin antibodies (IgM) (STEC HU antibody syndrome), ANA, anticentrom (scleroderma), plasma homocysteine levels, acid levels (Cobalamin C disease).

It is important to initiate treatment with Before starting the result of ADAMTS13 act should be started pending the result.

Provided that the ADAMTS13 activity i features are compatible with a diagnosis o started. Therapy with eculizumab is initiated weekly for the first 4 weeks, and then beg therapy every other week at a dose of 1200n Dose adjustment should be considered for pa (Alexion; Soliris® leaflet) [8].

If subsequent investigations show tha condition apart from aHUS, then eculizumab genetic investigations are available within sev

The markers of an active TMA resp eculizumab in virtually all patients wi abnormality. When patients exhibit a po treatment should be extended (chronic) as ac sheet (Alexion) [3]. Although, there is no rec appropriate duration of treatment, one stud discontinuing eculizumab therapy. During months, 3 of the ten patients experienc continuation, but then immediately resur recovered. Strict home monitoring for early aHUS is recommended [29].

In aHUS, whether renal function returr irreversible renal damage sustained before th renal function can take several months. The stopped early in TMA induced dialysis-dep point for terminate eculizumab is not clear should be taken into consideration. If ecul patient TMA markers (decrease of platelet creatinine >25%) should be monitored clos recurrent extra-renal TMA then eculizumab s

Immun treatment i in these cas

Althou evaluation levels of a patients. H allow for a recurrence

In pati genetic ana

Women during treat data on exp human plac complemen Therefore, needed. It i many medi and becaus breast-feedi after treatm

As alre cases/millio rates in adu patients in every age c accordingly prescribed u

Neverth long term ir possible inf patients and

1. Niche-Product

The total amount of health costs is tremendously high for some countries when it depends on the Gross National Product. Therefore a fair distribution is sometimes difficult to achieve.

On which grounds an individual patient has access to medication is determined by common morality which the national government of individual countries may have accomplished. Nation-states frequently claim special moral prerogatives to regulate health care and distribute health care resources.

Several ethical ways of thinking are put forward in the medical context. As a rule two philosophies are most common in biomedical ethics:

On one hand the principle of utilitarianism. Its major ethical element is consequentialism, the view that the rightness and goodness of any action depends solely on the goodness of the overall state of affairs consequent upon it. An act is morally right if it produces maximal benefit for the largest group. This means in the particular case of aHUS, that treatment should be available to every patient, who has clinical benefit from the medication with improvement of the prognosis;

On the other hand is the philosophy of communitarianism. In this kind of moral thought, the community or the state, rather than the individual, is the centre of any value system. Not the self-interest of an individual, but the global community should benefit from it. In case of the aHUS this may imply, that eculizumab can be reserved for young people with high life-expectancy instead of the elderly. In the future, young, active persons can get the money back, which were the costs for the community to treat them.

In practice, the different health care departments compromise between both ideas. The compromise reflects the reimbursement criteria.

On the other side of the medical field, the pharmaceutical industry has a patency on the drug and therefore power over the negotiation procedures. Both industry and governmental health care departments have to come to an optimal agreement to serve all patients in a win-win operation for each, which is what the communitarianist position recommends.

2. Genetic Screening

Progress in medical science and technology has had remarkable results in medical treatment and in underlying causes of several diseases, as well.

The rapidly expanding knowledge of human genetics and the exploration of heritable diseases, diagnosed by simple, but often expensive genetic tests can be prescribed to at least forestall or limit the effects of the disease. In the case of aHUS, it is known that detectable underlying mutations can be a reason for this disease.

Instead it is also known that genetic screening in the case of aHUS can exclude some patients from treatment of eculizumab, because of the uselessness of the therapy for them. Mutations in the DGKE gene for example, encoding diacylglycerol kinase epsilon (DKGE) has been postulated as responsibility for the development of a TMA.

This form of aHUS usually presents in the first year of life and does not respond to eculizumab. The mutations in DKGE are homozygous or heterozygous and when such a mutation is found in the absence of any mutations in complement genes, eculizumab should be withdrawn [28].

Screening is not only necessary to determine the real diagnosis, but familial screening is necessary when a suitable kidney donor is available.

However, (genetic) screening always confronts the persons involved with a moral dilemma. Firstly, genetic screening - if indicated - should be voluntary. An important implication of genetic screening is the ownership of the DNA and the results of the examination.

Secondly, reflections regarding ownership can be encapsulated in what one may term 'the principle of ownership'. Ownership is derived from permission; it is constituted within the morality of mutual respect. In one respect, claims to ownership are made insofar as the entity owned has been brought within the sphere of the owner, and as such violating that ownership would be a violation of the person of the owner.

Ownership claims by societies are just as difficult to establish as those by individuals; indeed, they are more difficult being that there is more involved. Things are owned insofar as they are the products of persons. There are three sorts of property: individual, communal (or social) and general.

Ownership can be registered by implied contract. This means the ownership exists of oneself, apart from explicit rules. Every person is the owner of his/her own (individual) DNA. However, human DNA is universal, which means the United Nations can claim the ownership of DNA as mutual (general) human property.

Ownership can also be recorded by explicit contract or consent. Such modes of ownership derive from formal procedures for agreeing to provide services or a product. In this situation, screening for aHUS is only allowed after written informed consent.

When the results of the screening are available a new ethical problem arises: who is the owner of these results? Because of the high potential for diagnostic and therapeutic purposes, researchers claim the intellectual ownership. These results have to be stored in a bio-bank and used for other research in the medical field, which means in the future it may well concern perhaps other patient populations. The benefits should be shared with other patients in general if it leads to benefit for other patient groups.

Therefore, funds may be collected by taxation to be distributed to all persons insofar as such possession by some fails to leave like material available for others to possess.

Such taxes are best collected internationally and should be paid not only by individuals and corporations, but by governments as well. Tax may also be collected as a charge for services [30].

3. Infectious Complications by *Neisseria*

The main adverse effect of eculizumab is an increased susceptibility to meningococcal infection due to the inhibition of the complement system's membrane-attack complex. According to the medication guide of the US Food and Drug Administration, a tetravalent unconjugated polysaccharide vaccine (serogroups A, C, Y, W135) has to be provided at least 2 weeks before the first dose of eculizumab. However, the advised vaccination only offers limited protection, because the most prevalent serogroup B meningococcal disease in European children is not included in the vaccine.

Therefore, penicillin prophylaxis should not only be considered, but also strongly advised to patients treated with eculizumab. The best strategy depends on the distribution of meningococcal serogroups and the availability of vaccines in different countries [31].

Patients less than two years old and those treated less than two weeks after receiving a meningococcal vaccine must receive treatment with appropriate prophylactic antibiotics until 2 weeks after vaccination. Revaccination could be possible according to the current medical guidelines (Alexion; Soliris® leaflet). A disadvantage of the 14-days pre-existing vaccination administration is the delay in starting Eculizumab treatment. In very urgent situations of aHUS manifestations, the pro and cons of eculizumab administration prior to vaccination, but additionally covered by penicillin should be balanced.

4. Quality of Life

In terms of health-related quality of life (HR-QoL), a significant increase from baseline in the mean EuroQoL group 5-dimension Self-Report Questionnaire (EQ-5D) score (the score ranges from 0 - 1) was reported in eculizumab recipients at week 26 and in the extension phase in two clinical trials. Both patient groups have renal damage, with or without renal replacement therapy.

A clinically meaningful EQ-5D score of 0.06 was exceeded by 80% of eculizumab recipients at week 26 and by 87% of eculizumab recipients after a median treatment duration of 64 weeks (trial 1), and 73% of patients in trial 2 throughout the treatment period [20, 32].

The EQ-5D is a standardized health questionnaire with 5 different health-care dimensions; e.g., mobility, self-care, activities in daily life, pain/discomfort, and feelings of unhappiness/depression; and is complementary to other Quality of Life measurement instruments, like SF-36. Particular organ specific QoL questionnaires are also available, like KDQOL (Kidney disease Quality of Life) for patients with renal replacement therapy. Although very few trials of QoL available for eculizumab in aHUS show a quality of life related benefit, it seems obvious, however, that further research in this field over long-term treatment is necessary. Side-effects of possible complications in long-term treatment are not known and different measurements should be taken at several different time-points.

Conclusion

The administration of Soliris® has serious advantages for a patient's personal life in particular and societies interest in general. No doubt eculizumab, if indicated, renders prognostic benefits. However, long-term side effects of eculizumab are still unknown. Frequently, medical screening for oncological manifestations should be carried out.

And a research field of interest should be the evolution of treatment, because although it has not yet been demonstrated, the possibility of developing anti-eculizumab antibodies cannot be excluded.

provided rationale for investigation of other indications, such as aHUS in which complement plays a role [19].

The safety profile of eculizumab for patients with aHUS was generally consistent with that in a study involving patients with paroxysmal nocturnal hemoglobinuria who received treatment for up to 8 years [22].

The efficacy and safety of eculizumab as a treatment for aHUS was evaluated in two prospective studies, and the response to eculizumab was similar between patients with mutations and/or anti-FH antibodies and those with no genetic abnormalities. The response was also similar regardless of the type of mutation identified. After six months of treatment with eculizumab, rates of hematological normalization reached 76% in resistant cases and 90% in chronic cases. Eculizumab was associated with significant increases in the estimated glomerular filtration rate (eGFR).

Earlier intervention with eculizumab was associated with significantly greater improvement in the eGFR. Eculizumab was also associated with improvement in health-related quality of life. No cumulative toxicity of therapy or serious infection-related adverse events, including meningococcal infections, were observed through the extension period.

After one year of eculizumab treatment, proteinuria levels were significantly lower than baseline values. Adverse side effects were peritonitis, influenza infection, venous disorder and severe hypertension.

Except for severe hypertension (this patient was already known with hypertension) all adverse events were possibly or probably drug-related. All serious adverse events possibly or probably related to eculizumab resolved without interruption of treatment.

Adverse events were similar among patient subgroups, including the patients who had undergone kidney transplantation and were receiving concomitant immunosuppressive therapy. Eculizumab increases the risk of infection by *Neisseria Meningitidis,* which prompted the vaccination of all patients against *Neisseria* before starting treatment or antibiotic prophylaxis, with no cases of meningitis produced. Survival was 100% [3, 20].

In a French retrospective study of adult patients with aHUS receiving eculizumab, 4 or more weekly 900 mg infusions, the risk of reaching ESRD within 3 months and 1 year of aHUS onset were reduced by half in eculizumab-treated patients compared with recent historical controls [21].

Several cases with other diseases or rare manifestations of aHUS and positive results after eculizumab treatment already have been published [23-26]. Knowledge of the use of eculizumab preventing or treating aHUS in the post-transplant settings, according to individualized recurrence risk assessment is limited. One prospective study followed 22 renal transplant recipients with aHUS who received off-label therapy with anti-C5. Nine patients, all carrying a complement genetic abnormality associated with a high risk of aHUS recurrence, received prophylactic eculizumab to prevent post-transplant recurrence. Eight of them had a successful recurrence-free post-transplant course and achieved a satisfactory graft function, while the remaining patient experienced early arterial thrombosis of the graft.

Thirteen renal transplant recipients were given eculizumab for post-transplant aHUS recurrence. A complete reversal of aHUS activity was obtained in all of them. Importantly, the delay of eculizumab initiation after the onset of the aHUS episode inversely correlated with the degree of renal function improvement. The patients in whom anti-C5 was subsequently stopped experienced a relapse. These data suggest that long-term eculizumab is highly effective for preventing and treating post-transplant aHUS recurrence and indicates that treatment with anti-C5 should be promptly started if a recurrence occurs [27]. Whether it will be safe to withdraw eculizumab in these patients after several years is not yet known.

Treatment

Early and intensive PE should be administrated until eculizumab is an available option. PE and FFP should be preferentially evaluated (1.5 per volume plasma (60 - 75ml/kg) per session. Sessions should be continued until platelet levels have normalized, hemolysis has stopped and a sustained improvement in renal function has been observed for several days. Later (sessions/week should be administered during the following 2 weeks, followed by another two weeks of 3 sessions per week and an individualized assessment for considering the appropriateness of continued treatment [3].

Prior to this point, it is necessary to vaccinate all patients against *Neisseria meningitides*. (Preferably with conjugated tetravalent vaccines against serotypes A, C, Y and W135).

In case that treatment with eculizumab cannot be delayed until obtaining vaccination, treatment can still be started along with antibiotic prophylaxis against *Neisseria meningitides*. In pediatric patients, vaccination against *Haemophilus influenza* and pneumococci is also necessary [3].

When a patient presents with features compatible with a diagnosis of aHUS, the following investigations should be undertaken to exclude other causes of a TMA: ADAMTS13 activity (TTP), stool culture, Shiga toxin, E. coli endotoxin antibodies (IgM) (STEC HUS), (HIV), AL antibody (APL antibody syndrome), ANA, anticentromere antibodies, Anti-ACL-70 (scleroderma), plasma homocysteine levels, plasma and urine methylmalonic acid levels (Cobalamin C disease).

It is important to initiate treatment with eculizumab as soon as possible. Before starting the result of ADAMTS13 activity should be available and PE should be started pending the result.

Provided that the ADAMTS13 activity is not <10% and that the clinical features are compatible with a diagnosis of aHUS, eculizumab should be started. Therapy with eculizumab is initiated intravenously at a dose of 900mg weekly for the first 4 weeks, and then beginning on week 5 maintenance therapy every other week at a dose of 1200mg intravenously is administered. Dose adjustment should be considered for patients with a body weight <40kg (Alexion; Soliris® leaflet) [8].

If subsequent investigations show that the TMA is due to another condition apart from aHUS, then eculizumab is withdrawn. The results of the genetic investigations are available within several weeks [28].

The markers of an active TMA respond rapidly to treatment with eculizumab in virtually all patients with an underlying complement abnormality. When patients exhibit a positive response to eculizumab, treatment should be extended (chronic) as advised by the drug technical data sheet (Alexion) [3]. Although, there is no recommendation regarding the most appropriate duration of treatment, one study experienced the possibility of discontinuing eculizumab therapy. During a cumulative observation of 95 months, 3 of the ten patients experienced relapse within 6 weeks of continuation, but then immediately resumed treatment and completely recovered. Strict home monitoring for early signs of relapse in patients with aHUS is recommended [29].

In aHUS, whether renal function returns is dependent on the extent of irreversible renal damage sustained before the onset of treatment. Recovery of renal function can take several months. Therefore, eculizumab should not be stopped early in TMA induced dialysis-dependent patients. Although, time-point for terminate eculizumab is not clear cut, a period of at least 4 months should be taken into consideration. If eculizumab is withdrawn in such a patient TMA markers (decrease of platelet count >25%, increase in serum creatinine >25%) should be monitored closely. If there is any evidence of recurrent extra-renal TMA then eculizumab should be restituted [28].

Immunosuppression therapy should be administrated as a concomitant treatment in patients with aHUS anti-FH antibodies. The response to treatment in these cases should be monitored through the evolution of antibody titres [3].

Although not necessary for the clinical diagnosis of aHUS, a complete evaluation of the complement system is recommended, including plasma levels of all complement factors and a complete genetic analysis of affected patients. However, a genetic diagnosis of abnormal complement genes would allow for assessing prognosis on an individual basis, as well as the risk of recurrence of the disease, making this a recommended step for all patients.

In patients who are potential candidates for kidney transplantation, the genetic analysis is indispensable [3].

Women of childbearing potential have to use effective contraception during treatment and up to 5 months after treatment. For Soliris®, no clinical data on exposed pregnancies are available. Human IgG are known to cross the human placental barrier, and thus eculizumab may potentially cause terminal complement inhibition in the fetal circulation and causes fetal morbidity. Therefore, Soliris® should be given to a pregnant woman only if clearly needed. It is unknown whether eculizumab is excreted into human milk. Since many medical products and immunoglobulins are secreted into human milk, and because of the potential for serious adverse reactions in nursing infants, breast-feeding should be discontinued during treatment and up to 5 months after treatment (Alexion; Soliris® leaflet).

Ethical Annotation

As already written above, aHUS has an annual incidence rate of 1 - 3 cases/million inhabitants' individuals younger than 18 years of age, with lower rates in adults. This means, aHUS is considered to be a rare disease, affecting patients in different age categories but adequate treatment is available for every age category. The drug eculizumab, is a product of niche marketing and accordingly very expensive. Eculizumab is not available to everyone and is prescribed under strict recommendation.

Nevertheless, eculizumab is a young drug and therefore information of long term intake and the achievable adverse events are still not available. The possible infectious complications by *Neisseria*, and the genetic screening for patients and their relatives needs further ethical investigation.

1. Niche-Product

The total amount of health costs is tremendously high for some countries when it depends on the Gross National Product. Therefore a fair distribution is sometimes difficult to achieve.

On which grounds an individual patient has access to medication is determined by common morality which the national government of individual countries may have accomplished. Nation-states frequently claim special moral prerogatives to regulate health care and distribute health care resources.

Several ethical ways of thinking are put forward in the medical context. As a rule two philosophies are most common in biomedical ethics:

On one hand the principle of utilitarianism. Its major ethical element is consequentialism, the view that the rightness and goodness of any action depends solely on the goodness of the overall state of affairs consequent upon it. An act is morally right if it produces maximal benefit for the largest group. This means in the particular case of aHUS, that treatment should be available to every patient, who has clinical benefit from the medication with improvement of the prognosis;

On the other hand is the philosophy of communitarianism. In this kind of moral thought, the community or the state, rather than the individual, is the centre of any value system. Not the self-interest of an individual, but the global community should benefit from it. In case of the aHUS this may imply, that eculizumab can be reserved for young people with high life-expectancy instead of the elderly. In the future, young, active persons can get the money back, which were the costs for the community to treat them.

In practice, the different health care departments compromise between both ideas. The compromise reflects the reimbursement criteria.

On the other side of the medical field, the pharmaceutical industry has a patency on the drug and therefore power over the negotiation procedures. Both industry and governmental health care departments have to come to an optimal agreement to serve all patients in a win-win operation for each, which is what the communitarianist position recommends.

2. Genetic Screening

Progress in medical science and technology has had remarkable results in medical treatment and in underlying causes of several diseases, as well.

The rapidly expanding knowledge of human genetics and the exploration of heritable diseases, diagnosed by simple, but often expensive genetic tests can be prescribed to at least forestall or limit the effects of the disease. In the case of aHUS, it is known that detectable underlying mutations can be a reason for this disease.

Instead it is also known that genetic screening in the case of aHUS can exclude some patients from treatment of eculizumab, because of the uselessness of the therapy for them. Mutations in the DGKE gene for example, encoding diacylglycerol kinase epsilon (DKGE) has been postulated as responsibility for the development of a TMA.

This form of aHUS usually presents in the first year of life and does not respond to eculizumab. The mutations in DKGE are homozygous or heterozygous and when such a mutation is found in the absence of any mutations in complement genes, eculizumab should be withdrawn [28].

Screening is not only necessary to determine the real diagnosis, but familial screening is necessary when a suitable kidney donor is available.

However, (genetic) screening always confronts the persons involved with a moral dilemma. Firstly, genetic screening - if indicated - should be voluntary. An important implication of genetic screening is the ownership of the DNA and the results of the examination.

Secondly, reflections regarding ownership can be encapsulated in what one may term 'the principle of ownership'. Ownership is derived from permission; it is constituted within the morality of mutual respect. In one respect, claims to ownership are made insofar as the entity owned has been brought within the sphere of the owner, and as such violating that ownership would be a violation of the person of the owner.

Ownership claims by societies are just as difficult to establish as those by individuals; indeed, they are more difficult being that there is more involved. Things are owned insofar as they are the products of persons. There are three sorts of property: individual, communal (or social) and general.

Ownership can be registered by implied contract. This means the ownership exists of oneself, apart from explicit rules. Every person is the owner of his/her own (individual) DNA. However, human DNA is universal, which means the United Nations can claim the ownership of DNA as mutual (general) human property.

Ownership can also be recorded by explicit contract or consent. Such modes of ownership derive from formal procedures for agreeing to provide services or a product. In this situation, screening for aHUS is only allowed after written informed consent.

When the results of the screening are available a new ethical problem arises: who is the owner of these results? Because of the high potential for diagnostic and therapeutic purposes, researchers claim the intellectual ownership. These results have to be stored in a bio-bank and used for other research in the medical field, which means in the future it may well concern perhaps other patient populations. The benefits should be shared with other patients in general if it leads to benefit for other patient groups.

Therefore, funds may be collected by taxation to be distributed to all persons insofar as such possession by some fails to leave like material available for others to possess.

Such taxes are best collected internationally and should be paid not only by individuals and corporations, but by governments as well. Tax may also be collected as a charge for services [30].

3. Infectious Complications by *Neisseria*

The main adverse effect of eculizumab is an increased susceptibility to meningococcal infection due to the inhibition of the complement system's membrane-attack complex. According to the medication guide of the US Food and Drug Administration, a tetravalent unconjugated polysaccharide vaccine (serogroups A, C, Y, W135) has to be provided at least 2 weeks before the first dose of eculizumab. However, the advised vaccination only offers limited protection, because the most prevalent serogroup B meningococcal disease in European children is not included in the vaccine.

Therefore, penicillin prophylaxis should not only be considered, but also strongly advised to patients treated with eculizumab. The best strategy depends on the distribution of meningococcal serogroups and the availability of vaccines in different countries [31].

Patients less than two years old and those treated less than two weeks after receiving a meningococcal vaccine must receive treatment with appropriate prophylactic antibiotics until 2 weeks after vaccination. Revaccination could be possible according to the current medical guidelines (Alexion; Soliris® leaflet). A disadvantage of the 14-days pre-existing vaccination administration is the delay in starting Eculizumab treatment. In very urgent situations of aHUS manifestations, the pro and cons of eculizumab administration prior to vaccination, but additionally covered by penicillin should be balanced.

4. Quality of Life

In terms of health-related quality of life (HR-QoL), a significant increase from baseline in the mean EuroQoL group 5-dimension Self-Report Questionnaire (EQ-5D) score (the score ranges from 0 - 1) was reported in eculizumab recipients at week 26 and in the extension phase in two clinical trials. Both patient groups have renal damage, with or without renal replacement therapy.

A clinically meaningful EQ-5D score of 0.06 was exceeded by 80% of eculizumab recipients at week 26 and by 87% of eculizumab recipients after a median treatment duration of 64 weeks (trial 1), and 73% of patients in trial 2 throughout the treatment period [20, 32].

The EQ-5D is a standardized health questionnaire with 5 different health-care dimensions; e.g., mobility, self-care, activities in daily life, pain/discomfort, and feelings of unhappiness/depression; and is complementary to other Quality of Life measurement instruments, like SF-36. Particular organ specific QoL questionnaires are also available, like KDQOL (Kidney disease Quality of Life) for patients with renal replacement therapy. Although very few trials of QoL available for eculizumab in aHUS show a quality of life related benefit, it seems obvious, however, that further research in this field over long-term treatment is necessary. Side-effects of possible complications in long-term treatment are not known and different measurements should be taken at several different time-points.

Conclusion

The administration of Soliris® has serious advantages for a patient's personal life in particular and societies interest in general. No doubt eculizumab, if indicated, renders prognostic benefits. However, long-term side effects of eculizumab are still unknown. Frequently, medical screening for oncological manifestations should be carried out.

And a research field of interest should be the evolution of treatment, because although it has not yet been demonstrated, the possibility of developing anti-eculizumab antibodies cannot be excluded.

References

[1]   Noris, M., Remuzzi, G. Atypical hemolytic-uremic syndrome. *N. Engl. J. Med.* 2009; 361(17): 1676-1687.

[2]   Loirat, C., Frémeaux-Bacchi, V. Atypical haemolytic uremic syndrome. *Orphanet J. Rare Dis.* 2011;6:60.

[3]   Campistol, J. M., Arias, M., Ariceta, G., Blasco, M., Espinosa, M., Grinyó, J. M., Praga, M., et al. *Nefrologia* 2013;33(1):27-45.

[4]   Sethi, S., Fervenza, F. C. Membranoproliferative glomerulonephritis - a new look at an old entity. *N. Engl. J. Med.* 2012; 366(12): 1119-1131.

[5]   Loirat, C., Noris, M., Fremeaux-Bacchi, V. Complement and the atypical haemolytic uremic syndrome in children. *Pediatr. Nephrol.* 2008; 23(11): 1957-1972.

[6]   Kavanagh, D., Anderson, H. E. Interpretation of genetic variants of uncertain significance in atypical haemolytic uremic syndrome. *Kidney Int.* 2012; 81: 11-13.

[7]   Kavanagh, D., Goodship, T. H. J. Atypical haemolytic Uremic syndrome, genetic basis and clinical manifestations. *Hematology Am. Soc. Hematol. Educ. Program* 2011; 201: 15-20.

[8]   Cataland, S. R., Wu, H. M. How I treat: The clinical differentition and initial treatment of adult patients with atypical hemolytic uremic syndrome. *Blood* 2014;123(16):2478-84.

[9]   Noris, M., Caprioli, J., Bresin, E., Mossali, C., Pianetti, G., Gamba, Daina, E., et al. *Clin. J. Am. Soc. Nephrol.* 2010; 5:1844-1859.

[10]   Holers, V. M. The spectrum of complement alternative pathway-mediated diseases. *Immunol. Rev.* 2008; 223:300-316.

[11]   Fang, C. J., Richards, A., Liszewski, M. K., Kavanagh, D., Atkinson, J. R. *Br. J. Haematol.* 2008;143:336-348.

[12]   Kavanagh, D., Goodship, T. H. J., Richards, A. *British Medical Bulletin.* 2006; 77 and 78: 5-22.

[13]   Janssen van Doorn, K., Dirinck, E., Verpooten, G. A., Couttenye, M. M. Complement factor H mutation associated with membranoproliferative glomerulonephritis with transformation to atypical haemolytic uraemic syndrome. *Clin. Kidney J.* 2013;6(2):216-219.

[14]   Sinha, A., Gulati, A., Saini, S., Blanc, C., Gupta, Gurjar, B. S., Saini, H., et al. Prompt plasma exchanges and immunosuppressive treatment improves the outcomes of anti-factor H autantibody-associated hemolytic uremic syndrome in children. *KI* 2013;85:1151-1160.

[15] Zuber, J., Le quintrec, M., Sberro-Soussan, R., Loirat, C., Frémeaux-Bacchi, V., Legendre, C. New insights into postrenal transplant hemolytic syndrome. *Nat. Rev. Nephrol.* 2011; 7(1):23-35.

[16] Nester, C., Stewart, Z., Meyers, D., Jetton, J., Nair, R., Reed, A., Thomas, C., et al. *Clin. J. Am. Soc. Nephrol.* 2011;6(6):1488-1494.

[17] Saland, J. M., Ruggenenti, P., Remuzzi, G., and the Consensus Study Group. *J. Am. Soc. Nephrol.* 2009;20:940-949.

[18] Davin, J.-C., Groothoff, J., Gracchi, V., Bouts, A. *Pediatr. Nephrol.* 2011;26:1915-1916.

[19] Rother, R. P., Rollins, S. A., Mojcik, C. F., Brodsky, R. A., Bell, L. Discovery and development of the complement inhibitor eculizumab for the treatment of paroxysmal nocturnal hemoglobinuria. *Nature Biotechnology* 2007; 25(11):1256-1488.

[20] Legendre, C. M., Licht, C., Muus, P., Greenbaum, L. A., Babu, S., Bedrosian, C., Bingham, C., Cohen, D. J., Delmas, Y., Dougls, K., et al. Terminal complement inhibitor eculizumab in atypical haemolytic-uremic syndrome. *N. Engl. J. Med.* 2013; 68:2169-81.

[21] Fakhouri, F., Delmas, Y., Provot, F., Barbet, C., Karras, A., Makdasi, R., Courivaud, C., et al. Insights from the use in clinical practice of eculizumab in adult patients with atypical haemolytic uremic syndrome affecting the native kidneys: an analysis of 19 cases. *AJKD* 2014; 63 (1): 40-8.

[22] Kelly, R. J., Hill, A., Arnold, L. M., Brooksbank, G. L., Richards, S. J., Cullen, M., Mitchell, L. D., et al. Long-term treatment with eculizumab in paroxysmal nocturnal hemoglobinuria: sustained efficacy and improvement survival. *Blood* 2011; 117(25):6786-92.

[23] Rousset-Rouvière, C., Cailliez, M., Garaix, F., Bruno, D., Laurent, D., Tsimaratos, M. Rituximab fails where eculizumab restores renal function in C3nef-related DDD. *Peditatr. Nephrol.* 2014;29:1107-1111.

[24] Sànchez-Moreno, A., De la Cerda, F. Eculizumab in dense-deposit disease after renal transplantation. *Pediatr. Nephrol.* 2014; 29:1107-1111.

[25] Rosenblad, T., Rebetz, J., Johansson, M., Békàssy, Sartz, L., Karpman, D. Eculizumab treatment for rescue of renal function in IgA nephropathy. *Pediatr. Nephrol.* 2014 in press.

[26] Hu, H., Nagra, A., Haq, M. R., Gilbert, R. D. Eculizumab in atypical haemolytic uraemic syndrome with severe cardiac and neurological involvement. *Pediatr. Nephrol.* 2014; 29:1103-1106.

[27] Zuber, J., Le Quintrec, M., Krid, S., Bertoye, C., Gueuntin, V., Lahoche, A., Heyne, N., et al. Eculizumab for atypical Hemolytic Uremic Syndrome Recurrence in renal transplantation. *Am. J. Transplant.* 2012; 12(12):3337-54.

[28] Scully, M., Goodship, T. How I treat thrombotic thrombocytopenic purpura and atypical haemolytic uraemic syndrome. *BJH* 2014; 164 (6): 759-66.

[29] Ardissino, G., Testa, S. Possenti, I., Tel, F., Paglialonga, F., Salardi, S., Tedeschi, S., et al. Discontinuation of eculizumab maintenance treatment for atypical haemolytic uremic syndrome: a report of 10 cases. *Am. J. Kidney Dis.* 2014 in press.

[30] Engelhardt, Jr. H. T. *The foundations of bioethics.* Second edition. New York Oxford. Oxford University Press. 1996. Pg: 165-166.

[31] Bouts, A., Monnens, L., Davin, J.-L., Struijk, G., Spanjaard, L. Insufficient protection by Neisseria meningitides vaccination alone during eculizmab therapy. *Pediatr. Nephrol.* 2011; 26(10):1919-20.

[32] Keating, G. M. Eculizumab: A review of its use in atypical haemolytic uraemic syndrome. *Drugs* 2013;73:2053-2066.

In: Hemolytic Uremic Syndrome
Editors: Glenna Clayton

ISBN: 978-1-63463-227-0
© 2015 Nova Science Publishers, Inc.

Chapter IV

Hemolytic Uremic Syndrome: Overview and Update

Naglaa Michel Habib Keriakos[1*]
and Rami N. Khouzam[2]

[1]NSA Medical Laboratory, Egypt, (Nassseh S. Amin Medical Laboratory)
[2]Department of Medicine, Division of Cardiovascular Diseases,
Interventional Cardiology Fellowship, University of Tennessee Health
Science Center, Cardiac Catheterization Laboratory
Methodist University Hospital, Memphis, Tennessee, US

Abstract

HUS is defined by the triad of haemolytic anaemia, acute renal failure, and thrombocytopenia. It became a public health problem following the European outbreak of E. coli (O104:H4) gastroenteritis in 2011 [1].

The disease mainly affects children one to 10 years of age. It begins after an incubation period of 4 to 7 days with abrupt onset of bloody diarrhea and abdominal pain. Two to ten days later, microangiopathy, haemolytic anaemia, thrombocytopenia, and acute renal failure develop. HUS microangiopathy can involve almost any organ, but damage to

---

* Corresponding author: Email: knaglaa@hotmail.com.

kidneys and central nervous system cause the most severe clinical problems [2].

HUS is classified into three primary types: (1) HUS due to infections, often associated with diarrhea (D+HUS), with the rare exception of HUS due to a severe disseminated infection caused by Streptococcus; (2) HUS related to complement abnormalities, such HUS is also known as "atypical HUS" and is not diarrhea associated (D-HUS); and (3) HUS of unknown etiology that usually occurs in the course of systemic diseases or physiopathologic conditions such as pregnancy [3].

Hemolytic Uremic Syndrome (HUS) is defined as a triad of micro-angiopathic hemolytic anemia, acute renal failure, and thrombocytopenia. This term was first used by Gasser et al. in 1955.

HUS is Classified According to the Etiology into 3 Categories

1) HUS due to infection causing diarrhea (D+HUS): 90% of cases:
    E Coli O157:H7 is the most common cause of diarrhea associated HUS, other strains of E. coli were reported to cause HUS outbreaks (*E. coli* O103:H25 in Norway, E. coli (STEC) O104:H4 in Germany) [1]. The reservoir of E. coli is the intestinal tract of domestic animals, and it is usually transmitted by undercooked meat or unpasteurized milk [2]. The incidence of HUS after infectious diarrhea is 15% in case of E. coli O157:H7 and 25% in case of E. coli O104:H4 [3].

2) HUS due to complement abnormalities known as atypical HUS (aHUS): < 10% of cases:
    The alternate pathway is responsible for pathogenesis of this type of HUS. Several mutations have been identified in genes encoding for complement proteins; such mutations involve complement factor H (CFH), complement factor I (CFI), thrombomodulin (THBD). Other mutations include C3 and factor B.
    Autoantibodies for CFH were identified, more recently autoantibodies to CFI were detected [4].

3) HUS of unknown etiology that occurs with systemic diseases (e.g., scleroderma, systemic lupus erythematosus and antiphospholipid syndrome), malignancy or pathophysiologic conditions such as

pregnancy [4]. It could also be drug-induced (e.g., anti-neoplastic, antiplatelet, quinine, or immune-suppressives) [4, 5].

Epidemiology

HUS is a rare disease; the incidence of Shiga toxin associated hemolytic uremic syndrome (D+HUS) is different in various countries with tendency to be higher in colder countries. In Europe and North America the incidence is highest between ages 1-5 years, while in Argentina, the incidence is higher in younger age; 6 mo-4 years [6].

Symptoms

HUS primarily occurs in children one to 10 years of age with average incidence of 1-3 cases /100,000 yearly. HUS is the most common cause of renal failure in children. After an incubation period of 4-7 days, the patient starts to develop watery diarrhea which is followed 1-3 days later by bloody diarrhea and other gastrointestinal symptoms including abdominal cramps, nausea and vomiting. Symptoms of HUS start 2-10 days later as diarrhea improves, the onset may be sudden with pallor, abdominal pain, vomiting, dark urine, drowsiness and sometimes edema.

aHUS Symptoms

The age of onset of aHUS can be quite variable, but the majority of patients present during childhood. In a cohort of 46 children with aHUS, Sellier-Leclerc et al. recorded occurrence before age 2 of in 70% (32 cases) of children and presentation in the first 3 months of life in 17% (8 cases) of cases [7].

When aHUS occurs in adulthood, it is more common in women; this sex difference does not seem to happen in childhood aHUS.

In the majority of children (80%), the onset of aHUS is triggered by an infectious process, such as an upper respiratory tract infection, fever or gastroenteritis. Thus, diarrhea preceding the onset of HUS does not exclude aHUS [7].

The onset of aHUS can be sudden or insidious and children usually present with pallor, lethargy, and decreased urine output. The majority of the patients have severe hypertension. In about 20% of children, extra-renal manifestations, including central nervous system or cardiac involvement, are present [7].

Extrarenal Complications

Occur in 50% of cases, including;

Endocrinological: Pancreatitis and glucose intolerance.

Central Nervous System: Irritability, disorientation, seizures, reduced consciousness, as well as cerebral infarction that occurred in some cases proved by MRI.

Gastro Intestinal: Colonic necrosis and perforation [1] which rarely occurs in the first week. It usually occurs later in the course of the disease [2].

Pathogenesis

HUS due to Infection Causing Diarrhea (D+HUS)

Shiga toxins have AB5 molecular structure, composed of one enzymatically active A subunit (32 kDa) and five identical B subunits (7.7 kDa each) that mediate the attachment of the toxin (AB5) to neutral glycolipid receptor globotriaosylceramide (Gb3, or CD77) on the surface of host cells.

Gb3 is a glycosphingolipid which is expressed in the kidney, brain, liver, pancreas, heart, and hemopoetic cells.

Epithelial and endothelial cells in the kidneys and the central nervous system that are sensitive to the cytotoxic action of Shigatoxin, while human monocytes and macrophages are resistant or insensitive, even though they carry Gb3. Resistant cells generate soluble cytokines and chemokines like tumor necrosis factor alpha (TNF-α) and interleukin-1β (IL-1β) which results in increased susceptibility of endothelial cells to toxin. This is caused by increasing the expression of Gb3 and different leukocyte adhesion molecules to trigger cytotoxicity of the toxin. The host response factors play an important role in the development of hemorrhagic colitis and HUS through inducing vascular damage [8].

Shiga toxin producing E. coli infects the large intestine causing destruction of the brush border microvilli. The toxin crosses the gastrointestinal epithelium to the circulation where it is carried by blood cells; binding to a receptor that has much less affinity to shiga toxin than Gb3 receptors. When shiga toxin reaches an organ that has Gb3 receptors, it detaches form blood cells and binds to this tissue. After shiga toxin binds Gb3 (globotriaosyceramide) receptors it is endocytosed into the cell and transported via Golgi apparatus to the endoplasmic reticulum and finally into the cytoplasm, where it inactivates ribosomes (by specifically depurinating the 28S rRNA), leading to cessation of protein synthesis and cell death. Death and detachment of endothelial cells lead to exposure of the underlying thrombogenic tissues [3].

VEGF-A

VEGFs (Vascular Endothelial Growth Factors) are a group of proteins including placental-derived growth factor, VEGF-A, VEGF-B, VEGF-C, and VEGF-D.

VEGF-A promotes angiogenesis, it has isoforms which are named according to their number of amino acids, i.e., $VEGF_{121}$, $VEGF_{145}$, $VEGF_{165}$, $VEGF_{189}$, $VEGF_{206}$. The most biologically active VEGF-A isoform is $VEGF_{165}$, which predominantly signals through VEGF receptor 2 (VEGFR2) that seems to mediate almost all of the known cellular responses to VEGF [9].

Local reduction of VEGF within the kidney is sufficient to trigger the pathogenesis of thrombotic microangiopathy, this was proved by Eremina et al. when they used conditional gene targeting to delete VEGF from renal podocytes in adult mice, which resulted in severe thrombotic glomerular injury [10].

The role of VEGF-A in the pathogenesis of shigatoxin-associated hemolytic uremic syndrome requires further study.

Atypical HUS (aHUS)

The alternate pathway is continuously at low level of activity, with spontaneous hydrolysis of C3 in serum. This produces the anaphylatoxin, C3a, which is pro-inflammatory, and C3b, which can bind to the surface of cells. Deficiency of complement regulatory proteins of the alternate pathway as a result of mutations or autoantibodies leads to continuous generation of C3 and C5 convertases, which leads to the formation of the MAC (membrane attack complex). This uninhibited activation of the complement cascade at the site of vascular endothelium leads to cell injury and detachment with exposure of underlying thrombogenic tissues and thrombotic microangiopathy. Certain vascular beds (especially renal) are more prone to injury than others [5].

Regulatory mechanisms of alternate complement pathway include serum-based and cell-based factors which can inactivate C3b when it is produced. Serum-based factors include complement factor H (a plasma glycoprotein that plays an important role in the regulation of the alternative pathway of complement by controlling both spontaneous fluid phase C3 activation and its deposition on host cells) [5] and factor I (a serine proteinase that inhibits the formation of the alternative pathway C3 convertase (C3bBb) by inactivating cell-bound C3b through proteolytic cleavage to iC3b). The cell-based receptors include CD46 (membrane cofactor protein) and thrombomodulin (THBD). Mutations in all these regulatory molecules have been described in patients with atypical hemolytic uremic syndrome [3].

Factor H mutations can be classified into 2 groups; one mutation that leads to low level of CFH (type I) and this is associated with low level of plasma C3, the other group leads to hypofunctional CFH (type II) and this is associated with normal plasma level of CFH and C3. More than 70 mutations of CFH have been identified. CFH mutations are found in 20%-30% of aHUS cases.

Factor I mutations (about 40 mutations have been found); either result in decreased production in factor I, or modification in protein structure which leads to decreased function.

MCP mutations, more than 40 mutations are detected in patients with aHUS, mutated MCP binds weakly to C3 and its function as a cofactor is lost. MCP mutations account for 5%-15% of aHUS. C3 plasma level is usually within normal, if lower than normal other associated complement factors mutations should be suspected [4].

Thrombomodulin mutations are found in 3-5% of cases of aHUS.,Mutated forms of THBD are less capable of deactivations of C3b.

Mutations in Factor B (CFB) and C3 are found in 1-4% of cases and 2-10% of cases of aHUS respectively. A rare form of aHUS complicates an inherited defect of intracellular cobalamin 1 (Cbl) metabolism [4].

Complement might also have a potential role in the pathogenesis of D+HUS. The first evidence for a role of the alternative complement pathway in shigatoxin-associated hemolytic uremic syndrome was the observation that affected patients who have low serum C3, high C3d (breakdown product of C3), high plasma Bb, and soluble C5b-9. Orth et al. showed that purified shigatoxin 2 can bind to the regulatory protein, complement factor H. This does not affect the ability of CFH to regulate the alternative complement pathway in the fluid/serum phase but decreases its ability to bind to cell membranes and prevent complement attack. This suggests that acquired complement dysfunction can occur as a result of shigatoxin effect which leads to uncontrolled complement activation contributing to disease process [3].

Patients with D+HUS also show elevated plasma Bb and soluble C5b-9 fragments as reported by Thurman et al. [11]; this suggests complement activation in shigatoxin-associated hemolytic uremic syndrome. Levels returned to normal 28 days after hospital discharge. Other markers of complement activation in D+HUS were detected by Stahl et al. [12], as they reported C3 deposition on platelets and C3 and C9 deposits in particles derived from monocytes and platelets in patients with shigatoxin associated HUS [3].,

Diagnosis

Clinically, the constellation of microangiopathic hemolysis, thrombocytopenia and renal failure is suggestive of Hemolytic Uremic Syndrome.

Laboratory findings:

- Findings consistent with hemolysis including anemia with presence of fragmented red blood cells (Schistocytes) in the peripheral blood film, Serum Haptoglobin levels are very low or absent, and elevated Lactate dehydrogenase (LDH) level.
- Low platelet count (commonly less than 100,000/ UL).
- Elevated fibrin degradation products and D-dimers.
- Polymorphonuclear leukocytosis.
- PT and aPTT are usually normal or minimally prolonged.
- BUN and creatinine are quite high.
- Urine contains hemoglobin, hemosiderin, albumin, and microscopically: RBCs, WBCs and casts.

Enterohemorrhagic E. coli (EHEC) Diagnosis

EHEC infection can cause HUS even without diarrhea.

EHEC urinary tract infection can induce HUS which suggests the need to perform microscopic examination and culture of urine sample. Family history should be taken and knowledge about epidemic infections in the area is a very helpful diagnostic tool. Stools should be collected and tested specifically for E. coli O157:H7 with culture, Polymerase Chain Reaction (PCR), serology and anti-O157-antibody titer in serum. PCR and testing for anti-LPS antibodies of prevalent serotypes of E. coli should be conducted [4].

Atypical HUS Diagnosis

- C3 level, if low this indicates complement dysregulation although normal C3 levels do not exclude dysregulation.
- Marker of terminal complement activation (membrane attack complex C5a-C9) level in blood is elevated [13].
- Factor H and Factor I plasma concentrations. Might be normal in case of mutations.
- Anti-factor H auto-antibodies should be measured.
- Mutation analysis of complement factors (Complement factor H, Membrane Cofactor Protein, Complement factor I, CFB and C3). In patients with aHUS mutations in factor H, factor I and MCP were detected.
- ADAMTS13 deficiency generally does not present as HUS but as thrombotic thrombocytopenic purpura (TTP) [4, 14]. A disintegrin and metalloprotease with thrombospondin type 1 motif, 13 (ADAMTS13) activity >10% is suggestive of HUS when patient is presenting with the triad of hemolytic anemia, thrombocytopenia and acute renal impairment [13].

Von Willebrand factor (vWF) is a glycoprotein, which is the carrier protein for the plasma coagulation protein factor VIII (F-VIII) and promotes platelet adhesion and subsequent aggregation at the sites of vascular damage. A disintegrin and metalloprotease with thromobospondin type I repeats 13 (ADAMTS-13) is discovered to be the vWF-cleaving (Von Willibrand Factor) protease. Recent studies showed that the deficiency or dysfunction of ADAMTS-13 could result in the survival of uncleaved or partially cleaved large vWF multimers and these were regarded as the major cause of idiopathic TTP [15].

Renal Biopsy

Fibrin deposition and polymorphonuclear infiltration of renal tissue is usually seen in hemolytic uremic syndrome [16].

Specific pathological findings in HUS patients with acute renal failure are glomerular microthrombi.

Treatment Options

Current management focuses on supportive therapy. Clinical care involves fluid and electrolyte balance, management of hypertension, nutritional support, and fluid and electrolyte replacement and renal dialysis if required. Understanding the pathogenesis of HUS better, may allow development of direct treatment strategy.

1. Antibiotics

Studies showed that the use of antibiotics, especially bactericidal antibiotics (beta-lactams, quinolones, aminoglycosides, nitroimidazoles and sulfa containing antibiotics) can increase the risk of development of HUS following verotoxigenic E. coli infection, quinolones in particular can increase verotoxin expression. The use of bacteriostatic antibiotics did not show any significant difference in risk of development of HUS. Antibiotics may increase the risk of the hemolytic–uremic syndrome by causing the release of Shiga toxin from injured bacteria in the intestine, making the toxin more available for absorption.

The use of fosfomycin, macrolides, and newer generations of carbapenems as effective therapy for prevention of HUS still needs further investigations, despite clinical improvement in patients on fosfomycin further more structured studies with control group are needed to support this. Routine use of antibiotics is not recommended [3,17].

2. Plasma Exchange

Plasma exchange is effective in atypical forms of hemolytic uremic syndrome. However, the use of plasma exchange in VTEC-induced (Verotoxigenic E coli) hemolytic uremic syndrome is less evidence-based. Plasma exchange is postulated to remove proinflammatory and prothrombotic factors [3].

In adults, because of the excellent results achieved in the treatment of TTP and difficulty in distinguishing HUS from TTP, therapy with plasmapheresis is often used [18].

Immunoadsorption achieves 85% removal of IgG compared with 40% in plasma exchange. Investigators showed that the neurological status of the patients improved noticeably following immunoadsorption [19].

3. Shiga Toxin Neutralizing Strategies

Shigatoxin binding by multivalent ligands leads to clearance via the reticuloendothelial system. A cell-permeable peptide with shigatoxin 2-binding properties (PPP-tet) was recently developed. This molecule had the additional benefit of diverting shigatoxin to lysosomal degradation instead of being transferred to the endoplasmic reticulum. Due to the cell-permeable nature of PPP-tet, it could potentially be effective even after binding of shigatoxin to the cell membrane and could have a wider therapeutic window in patients. This treatment rescued mice from lethal shigatoxigenic E. coli challenge when given orally at 3 days. In a primate animal model, PPP-tet also decreased the severity of kidney injury when given 24 hours after shigatoxin [3].

4. Complement Inhibitors and Eculizumab

Eculizumab is a recombinant humanized monoclonal antibody that binds to complement C5 protein, inhibiting its cleavage, and thus preventing the generation of the terminal complement attack complex C5b-9 [20]. Eculizumab appears to be a highly effective treatment for aHUS [21].

In total, 196 patients from nine German centers were treated with more than one dose of eculizumab. Majority of patients had severe cerebral and renal involvement requiring renal replacement therapy. After 8 weeks of treatment, 95% of patients showed a partial or complete improvement of hematological parameters and neurological complications. 56% had normal renal function while 36% remained dialysis-dependent. It is notable that this study included multiple concomitant treatments and was missing control groups; therefore it should be considered with caution [3].

5. Renal Transplantation

Cases of Shiga toxin induced HUS (D+HUS) rarely progress to end stage renal disease (ESRD), but when this happens, renal transplantation has good outcome with less than 10% recurrence rate. On the other hand, patients with aHUS have much higher rates of progressing to ESRD (more than 50%), and they usually have poor prognosis when renal transplantation is performed with more 50% recurrence rate and graft loss.

In a HUS, patients with factor H and factor I mutations have poor prognosis after renal transplantation with graft loss within the first 2 years (both factor H and factor I are produced by the live, a defect that persist as a predisposing factor for HUS even after renal transplantation). Patients with mutations in MCP seem to have better outcome as MCP is a transmembrane protein that is highly expressed in the kidney and transplantation of kidney that express normal MCP should correct the defect [4, 5].

In conclusion, renal transplantation is recommended for patients with D+ HUS, while among patients with aHUS only those who have MCP mutations have a good prognosis after renal transplantation. For other aHUS causes renal transplantation is not recommended. Generally renal transplantation from related living donor is not recommended [4].

Santos et al. stated that renal transplantation does not improve the 5 year survival in patients with HUS related renal failure; furthermore the graft outcome was worse in those who have HUS than recipients with other kidney disease. The rate of graft loss was higher in patients who had HUS recurrence after transplantation than those who didn't have recurrence. They retrospectively studied a US registry for the outcome of 323 kidney transplants in adults with HUS and of 121,311 transplants in adults with other renal diseases during the period 1999-2009 [22].

6. Combined Liver- Kidney Transplantation

This seems to be a promising option for treatment of patients with aHUS induced ESRD, when a HUS is due to CFH, or FI mutations. Number of cases studied is still few, but shows favorable outcomes when patients are treated with intensive plasma therapy before and during surgery [23, 24].

Prognosis

Several clinical and biochemical signs at onset of HUS have been suggested to be related to poor prognosis. Among the most important indicators of poor prognosis are leukocytosis and anuria. A case-control study from 2006 dealt with 17 deaths among patients with HUS (2 of the deaths were excluded due to treatment withdrawal due to their preexisting conditions) and concluded that patients who are admitted with oligoanuria, dehydration, WBC $> 20 \times 10^9$/L and haematocrit $> 23\%$, are at serious risk of fatal HUS [1, 25].

HUS is the most common cause of acute renal impairment in children, with 5% mortality and 25% chance of developing chronic renal disease or hypertension.

One report suggesting 50% recovery without long-term complications, in patients who have central nervous involvement in association with HUS, mortality rate is 17% and in another report 30% chance of long term neurological deficit [3].

Complement mediated HUS (aHUS) has a worse prognosis compared with shiga toxin mediated HUS, often resulting in end stage renal disease (50%-80%) and acute (aHUS) mortality rate of 8% [26]. In general, patients with aHUS have a poor prognosis. More than 60% of patients with mutations of CFH, CFI, C3, CFB and THBD (thrombomodulin) either die or develop ESRD within1 year of presentation. Patients with MCP have a better long-term outcome, with only 30% progressing to ESRD, though they tend to have a frequently relapsing course [4].

Conclusion

Hemolytic Uremic Syndrome (HUS) is a rare disease composed of a triad of microangiopathy, acute renal impairment, and thrombocytopenia. It mainly affects children younger than 10 years of age hence considered the most common cause of renal failure in children. HUS is frequently the result of infection with Shiga toxin producing bacteria (E coli). In recent years, studies regarding HUS have developed a better understanding of its pathophysiology. As a result, more diagnosis methods as well as treatment options have developed. Knowledge of HUS is increasing and further studies are conducted aiming at a better understanding leading to definitive and effective treatments of the disease.

References

[1]   Krogvold, L; Henrichsen, T; Bjerre, A; Brackman, D; Dollner, H; Gudmundsdottir, H; Syversen, G; Næss, PA; Bangstad, HJ. Clinical aspects of a nationwide epidemic of severe haemolytic uremic syndrome (HUS) in children. *Scand J Trauma Resusc Emerg Med*, 2011, 19, 44.

[2]   Hye, Jin Chang; Hwa, Young Kim; Jae, Hong Choi; Hyun, Jin Choi; Jae, Sung Ko; Il Soo, Ha; Hae, Il Cheong; Yong, Choi; Hee, Gyung Kang. Shiga toxin-associated hemolytic uremic syndrome complicated by intestinal perforation in a child with typical hemolytic uremic syndrome.,*Korean J Pediatr.*, 2014, 57(2), 96-99.

[3]   Keir, LS; Marks, SD; Kim, JJ. Shigatoxin associated hemolytic uremic syndrome: current molecular mechanisms and future therapies. *Drug des devel ther.*, 2012, 6, 195-208.

[4]   Salvadori, M; Bertoni, E. Update on hemolytic uremic syndrome: Diagnostic and therapeutic recommendations. *World J Nephrol.*, 2013, 2(3), 56–76.

[5]   Bresin, E; Daina, E; Noris, M; Castelletti, F; Stefanov, R; Hill, P; Goodship, THJ; Remuzzi, G. Outcome of Renal Transplantation in Patients with Non–Shiga Toxin–Associated Hemolytic Uremic Syndrome. Prognostic Significance of Genetic Background. *CJASN*, 2006, 1, 88-99.

[6]   Johnson, S; Mark, Taylor C. Hemolytic Uremic Syndrome. *Pediatric Nephrology*, 2009, 7, 1155–1180.

[7]   Joseph, C; Gattineni, J. Complement disorders and hemolytic uremic syndrome. *Current Opinion in Pediatrics*, 2013, 25(2), 209-215.
[8]   Moazzezy, N; Oloomi, M; Bouzari, S. Effect of Shiga Toxin and Its Subunits on Cytokine Induction in Different Cell Lines. *Int J Mol Cell Med.*, 2014, 3(2), 108–117.
[9]   Foster, RR. The Importance of Cellular VEGF Bioactivity in the Development of Glomerular Disease. *Nephron Experimental Nephrology*, 2009, 113, e8–e15.
[10] Eremina, V; Jefferson, JA; Kowalewska, J; Hochster, H; Haas, M;,Weisstuch, J; Richardson, C; Kopp, JB; Golam Kabir, M; Backx, PH; Gerber, HP; Ferrara, N; Barisoni, L; Alpers, CE; Quaggin, SE. VEGF inhibition and renal thrombotic microangiopathy. *N Engl J Med.*, 2008, 358, 1129–1136.
[11] Thurman, JM; Marians, R; Emlen, W; Wood, S; Smith, C; Akana, H; Holers, VM; Lesser, M; Kline, M; Hoffman, C; Christen, E; Trachtman, H. Alternative pathway of complement in children with diarrhea-associated hemolytic uremic syndrome. *Clin J Am Soc Nephrol.*, 2009, 4, 1920–1924.
[12] Ståhl, AL; Sartz, L; Karpman, D. Complement activation on platelet-leukocyte complexes and microparticles in enterohemorrhagic Escherichia coli-induced hemolytic uremic syndrome. *Blood*, 2011, 117, 5503–5513.
[13] Cataland, SR; Holers, VM; Geyer, S; Yang, S; Wu, HM. Biomarkers of terminal complement activation confirm the diagnosis of aHUS and differentiate aHUS from TTP. *Blood*, 2014, 123(24), 3733-3738.
[14] Ariceta, G; Besbas, N; Johnson, S; Karpman, D; Landau, D; Licht, C; Loirat, C; Pecoraro, C; Mark Taylor, C; Van de Kar, N; VandeWalle, J; Zimmerhackl, LB. Guideline for the investigation and initial therapy of diarrhea-negative hemolytic uremic syndrome. *Pediatr Nephrol.*, 2009, 24, 687–696.
[15] Feng, Yu; Ying, Tan; Ming-Hui, Zhao. Lupus nephritis combined with renal injury due to thrombotic thrombocytopaenic purpura-haemolytic uraemic syndrome. *Nephrol. Dial. Transplant*, 2010, 25(1), 145-152.
[16] Fallahzadeh, MA; Fallahzadeh, MK; Derakhshan, A; Shorafa, E; Mojtahedi, Y; Geramizadeh, B; Fallahzadeh, MH. A case of atypical hemolytic uremic syndrome. *Iran J Kidney Dis.*, 2014, 4, 341-343.
[17] Craig, S; Wong, MD; Srdjanjelacic, BS; Rebecca, L; Habeeb, BS; Sandra, L; Watkins, MD; Phillipi. Tarr, MD. The risk of hemolytic-

Uremic Syndrome after antibiotic treatment of E. Coli O157: H7 infections. *N Engl J Med.*, 2000, 342(26),1930-1936.

[18] Dundas, S; Murphy, J; Soutar, RL; Jones, GA; Hutchinson, SJ; Todd, WT. Effectiveness of therapeutic plasma exchange in the 1996 Lanarkshire Escherichia coli O157:H7 outbreak. *Lancet*, 1999, 354, 1327–1330.

[19] Greinacher, A; Friesecke, S; Abel, P; Dressel, A; Stracke, S; Fiene, M; Ernst, F; Selleng, K; Weissenborn, K; Schmidt, BM; Schiffer, M; Felix, SB; Lerch, MM; Kielstein, JT; Mayerle, J. Treatment of severe neurological deficits with IgG depletion through immunoadsorption in patients with Escherichia coli O104:H4-associated haemolytic uraemic syndrome: a prospective trial. *Lancet*, 2011, 378(9797), 1166-1173.

[20] Schmidtko, J; Peine, S; El-Housseini, Y; Pascual, M; Meier, P. Treatment of atypical hemolytic uremic syndrome and thrombotic microangiopathies: a focus on eculizumab. *Am J Kidney Dis.*, 2013, 61, 289-299.

[21] Rathbone, J; Kaltenthaler, E; Richards, A; Tappenden, P; Bessey, A; Cantrell, A. A systematic review of eculizumab for atypical haemolytic uraemic syndrome (aHUS). *BMJ open.*, 2013, 3(11), e003573.

[22] Santos, AH; Jr. Casey, MJ; Wen, X; Zendejas, I; Faldu, C; Rehman, S; Andreoni, KA. Outcome of kidney transplants for adults with hemolytic uremic syndrome in the U.S.: a ten-year database analysis. *Ann Transplant.*, 2014, 19, 353-361.

[23] Saland, JM; Ruggenenti, P; Remuzzi, G. Liver-kidney transplantation to cure atypical hemolytic uremic syndrome. *J Am Soc Nephrol.*, 2009, 20, 940–949.

[24] Jalanko, H; Peltonen, S; Koskinen, A; Puntila, J; Isoniemi, H; Holmberg, C; Pinomäki, A; Armstrong, E; Koivusalo, A; Tukiainen, E; et al. Successful liver-kidney transplantation in two children with aHUS caused by a mutation in complement factor H. *Am J Transplant.*, 2008, 8, 216–221.

[25] Oakes, RS; Siegler, RL; McReynolds, MA; Pysher, T; Pavia, AT. Predictors of, Fatality in postdiarrheal hemolytic uremic syndrome. *Pediatrics.*, 2006, 117, 1656-1662.,

[26] Posnik, B; Sikorska, D; Hoppe, K; Schwermer, K; Pawlaczyk, K; Oko, A. Acute Progression of Adult-Onset Atypical Hemolytic-Uremic Syndrome due to CFH Mutation: A Case Report. *Case Rep Nephrol.*, 2013, 2013, 739-820.

Index

J

K

L

M

S

scleroderma, 83, 94
sclerosis, 50
secrete, 8
secretion, 21, 52
segmental glomerulosclerosis, 50
sensitization, 59
sepsis, 11, 16, 26
serine, 98
serology, 100
serum, 13, 37, 38, 39, 40, 43, 47, 51, 55, 72, 83, 97, 98, 99, 100
sheep, 45, 48
Shiga toxin, vii, 2, 6, 7, 8, 9, 12, 21, 22, 34, 35, 83, 95, 96, 97, 101, 103, 105
shock, 67
showing, 5, 11
side effects, 81, 88
signalling, 21
signals, 12, 97
signs, 3, 83, 104
skin, 9
small intestine, 40
solution, viii, 30, 32, 36, 39, 48, 52, 59, 63
somatic cell, 78
somatic mutations, 80
specialists, 32
spinal cord, 23
spinal cord injury, 23
spontaneous recovery, 34
state(s), 2, 5, 6, 7, 8, 22, 24, 85
steroids, 35, 49, 53, 58, 59, 60
stimulation, 9, 12, 20, 47
stimulus, 5, 8
stomach, 50
stool culture, 83
Streptococcus, x, 94
stress, 7
stress response, 7
stroke, 11, 23
subgroups, 81
substitution, viii, 30, 33, 34, 39, 59, 60
substrate, 10, 16
sulfate, 4, 18

suppression, 25, 45, 47
survival, 16, 42, 49, 58, 60, 62, 90, 100, 103
survival rate, 42, 49, 62
susceptibility, 87, 96
symptoms, vii, 3, 13, 43, 50, 53, 77, 95
syndrome, vii, 2, 7, 9, 14, 21, 22, 27, 28, 33, 34, 35, 37, 38, 40, 42, 43, 47, 49, 52, 53, 60, 65, 66, 69, 70, 73, 76, 83, 89, 90, 91, 101, 102, 105, 106, 107
synthesis, 54, 55, 62
systemic lupus erythematosus, 31, 45, 94

T

T cell(s), 39, 60, 62
target, 2, 8, 26
techniques, viii, 29, 58
technology(s), viii, 30, 56, 85
testing, 17, 100
therapeutic apheresis, viii, 30, 39, 56, 58, 59, 62, 63, 64
therapeutic approaches, 13
therapeutic interventions, viii, 2, 58
therapeutic plasma exchange (TPE), viii, 30, 31, 32, 33, 34, 35, 36, 39, 40, 41, 42, 43, 44, 45, 48, 50, 51, 53, 54, 55, 59, 60, 61, 62, 63, 64, 66, 72, 107
therapeutics, 56
therapy, viii, ix, 10, 22, 30, 31, 32, 34, 35, 39, 40, 42, 44, 45, 46, 47, 48, 49, 50, 51, 52, 53, 56, 57, 59, 60, 61, 62, 63, 65, 68, 69, 70, 71, 76, 79, 80, 81, 82, 83, 84, 86, 91, 101, 102, 104, 106
therapy interventions, 34
thrombin, vii, 1, 2, 3, 4, 5, 6, 7, 8, 9, 10, 15, 16, 18, 20, 22, 23
thrombin activation, vii, 1, 2, 7, 16
thrombocyte, 49
thrombocytopenia, vii, x, 3, 9, 13, 34, 76, 93, 94, 99, 100, 105
thrombocytopenic purpura, 2, 17, 19, 22, 23, 24, 25, 26, 65, 91, 100
thrombomodulin, vii, 2, 4, 6, 10, 11, 12, 13, 15, 16, 18, 19, 20, 22, 23, 24, 25, 27, 28, 78, 94, 98, 104

U

V

W

Y